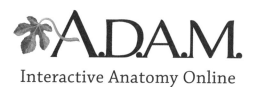

Interactive Anatomy Online

STUDENT LAB ACTIVITY GUIDE

FOURTH EDITION

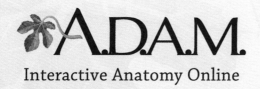

Interactive Anatomy Online

STUDENT LAB ACTIVITY GUIDE
FOURTH EDITION

SCOTT D. SCHAEFFER

Associate Professor of Biology, Harford Community College
Bel Air, Maryland

Wolters Kluwer | Lippincott Williams & Wilkins
Health

Philadelphia · Baltimore · New York · London
Buenos Aires · Hong Kong · Sydney · Tokyo

Publisher: Christopher Johnson
Acquisitions Editor: David Troy
Senior Product Manager: Amy Millholen
Production Product Manager: Marian Bellus
Design Coordinator: Stephen Druding
Marketing Manager: Sarah Schuessler
Compositor: SPi Global
Printer: RRD - Shenzhen

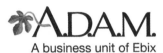

A business unit of Ebix

Printed in the People's Republic of China

Library of Congress Cataloging-in-Publication Data

Schaeffer, Scott D.
  A.D.A.M. Interactive Anatomy online : student lab activity guide / Scott D. Schaeffer. — 4th ed.
    p. ; cm.
  ADAM Interactive Anatomy online
  Rev. ed. of: A.D.A.M. Interactive Anatomy student lab guide / Mark Lafferty, Samuel Panella. 3rd ed. c2005.
  Includes bibliographical references and index.
  ISBN 978-1-4511-2039-4 (alk. paper)
  I. Lafferty, Mark. A.D.A.M. Interactive Anatomy student lab guide. II. Title. III. Title: ADAM Interactive Anatomy online.
  [DNLM: 1. Problems and Exercises—Laboratory Manuals. 2. Anatomy—Laboratory Manuals. QS 18.2]
  611.0076—dc23

                                                                                2012039437

About the Author

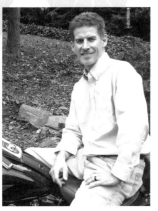

Scott D. Schaeffer earned a B.S. in health and physical education with an exercise science concentration from West Chester University in West Chester, Pennsylvania. He earned a D.C., magna cum laude, from Palmer College of Chiropractic in Davenport, Iowa, where he first experienced his love of teaching as a GTA in the human cadaver laboratory. For over a decade, Dr. Schaeffer has been inspiring his students in the classroom, injecting humor and real-world experience into his daily lessons.

Dr. Schaeffer is presently Associate Professor of Biology at Harford Community College in Bel Air, Maryland, where his primary responsibility is teaching Human Anatomy and Physiology to nursing and allied health students. He also regularly teaches The Human Body in Health and Disease, Nutrition, and Medical Terminology and Ethics. He enjoys watching students develop important critical thinking skills, believing it is easier to see what a student has learned by the questions they ask, rather than by the questions they answer. Dr. Schaeffer has served as A.D.A.M.'s primary Subject Matter Expert in the development of Anatomy and Health & Wellness web-based educational products. He also served as a Contributor and Content Reviewer for the following A.D.A.M. Education products: *A.D.A.M. Interactive Anatomy*, *A.D.A.M. Inside Out*, *A.D.A.M. Inside Out—Health & Wellness*, *A.D.A.M. Anatomy Practice*, and *A.D.A.M. Lab Exercises*.

Dr. Schaeffer is married with three children, two stepchildren, and a granddaughter. He and his wife, Gay, keep busy attending the school activities and sporting events of their children. In the warmer months, they enjoy motorcycling and try to log as many miles on their Harley as their hectic schedule allows. He also enjoys spending time in the kitchen and watching the Food Network and the Cooking Channel for tasty, new ideas.

A Note to Students

Dear Student,

Throughout my 9 years as a college student and another 14 years teaching college students, I have witnessed some big changes in education. Libraries seem to be less full as students now have access to mountains of information right from their smart phones. Textbooks are carried around less as eBooks put the same information at students' fingertips. Social media has made students adept at communicating in bytes as little as 140 characters or less. Instead of students sitting down and reading textbooks from beginning to end, as in days past, today's student learning preferences seem to be more visual and more interactive. Students prefer learning in short bursts, using multiple modalities.

A.D.A.M. Interactive Anatomy Online: Student Lab Activity Guide has been redesigned with the needs of today's student in mind. When studying human anatomy and physiology, it is the physiology that really ties things together. The physiology ultimately brings anatomy to life and helps it make sense. When it comes right down to it, anatomy is just a lot of memorization. As if that isn't boring enough, it is often the memorization of some very strange terms. In fact, I have heard some students liken the study of anatomy to that of a foreign language. The fourth edition of *A.D.A.M. Interactive Anatomy Online: Student Lab Activity Guide* has been completely revamped in an effort to make the study of human anatomy more meaningful, applicable, and dare I say exciting.

Each chapter begins with a short introduction to the organ system. A bit of background information has been added to each chapter in an effort to make the subject matter more meaningful. Important terms are found in bold throughout the text and help key you in on concepts critical to the application of human anatomy. Each chapter is subdivided into smaller, more manageable Lab Activities. Instead of sitting down to tackle an entire chapter in one sitting, the smaller Lab Activity sections allow you to learn the subject matter in chunks. This allows for the mastery of one subject before progression to the next. It also allows you to hone in on what material you find most challenging and easily go back to that area for review.

Clinical Applications boxes have been added to the new edition in an attempt to bring the material to life. Strict memorization tends to be somewhat difficult. The ability to understand and actually see why the material is important, that is, "when will I use this in the real world?" tends to make the subject matter more meaningful. Each chapter introduces at least a few clinically based examples to further engage you in active learning and let you develop your critical thinking skills.

New to this edition is the introduction of beautiful four-color images hand selected from the 30,000-plus images in the *A.D.A.M. Interactive Anatomy* (A.I.A.) image bank. One of the biggest challenges I have seen in the lab setting, as an instructor, is the manner in which many texts identify structures found within images using "leader lines." It is not uncommon for an image to have as many as five or six lines pointing to various places on the same organ. So which line is which? In an effort to make this guide more interactive, I have opted to present all of the images cleanly, without the use of leader lines. The purpose is twofold: First, it allows you to draw in the appropriate lines based on what your instructor decides are the most appropriate features for you to recognize. What is deemed appropriate for one class setting may not be appropriate for another. Secondly, in order to retain all of these new terms beyond what is simply needed to pass the test, you need to do more than just memorize a list of terms. Not only do the images in this guide allow for the addition of your own leader lines, but there is also adequate room for you to write in the appropriate terms and label your lines. In the allied health field, spelling is absolutely crucial! Take a look at some of the medications that are out there. It is not enough to simply say "I think it starts with a V—can I have partial credit?" There may be 20-plus medications that start with a "V" and if you "can't remember" or "guess" when spelling in the patient's chart, it can lead to big problems for everyone involved. In health care, the misplacing of a decimal, sloppy handwriting, and misspelled words can have dire consequences for your patients. There is little that would make an attorney for the plaintiff happier than to project your handwritten patient notes on an 8-foot screen in the courtroom pointing out all of your misspellings. I can hear them say, "If this 'health care provider' is so sloppy with their charting, can you imagine how sloppy their care must be?" SPELLING COUNTS! To that end, I felt it most appropriate to give you the opportunity to hone your skills by writing in your own labels on the images.

Keep in mind that I picked the images I felt best represented the most appropriate views for labeling a majority of structures. Because the image library within A.I.A. is so large, there may be images not found in this guide but available in A.I.A., which show better renditions of particular features. While this text was written to serve as a "stand-alone" text, student access to the online A.I.A. program allows for a more in-depth immersion in A&P. When possible, you will notice in the guide that you are directed to alternate images within A.I.A. for you to explore different views of some subject matter. I encourage you to do your own exploration as you develop your unique areas of interest. Use the Dissectible Anatomy feature to peel back layer-by-layer views of the body. Click on Clinical Animations or Clinical Illustrations to enhance your working knowledge of the material. Explore the built-in Encyclopedia function to help drive these ideas home and tie the laboratory information together with the material presented in the lecture.

It is my most sincere hope that using this guide as it was designed will place you on the path to mastery of human anatomy and physiology. The added background information, use of Clinical Applications boxes, clean color images, and tailored review exercises have been designed with the purposeful intent of making the study of A&P as meaningful and efficient as possible for you, the student.

—Scott Schaeffer

Preface

ABOUT *A.D.A.M. INTERACTIVE ANATOMY ONLINE: STUDENT LAB ACTIVITY GUIDE*

The latest edition of *A.D.A.M. Interactive Anatomy Online: Student Lab Activity Guide* has been dramatically redesigned in an effort to facilitate student learning while allowing for instructor flexibility in the classroom/laboratory setting. *A.D.A.M. Interactive Anatomy Online: Student Lab Activity Guide* is written for those students in introductory human anatomy and physiology courses preparing for a career in a variety of allied health disciplines. This lab guide is designed as a stand-alone text, containing all of the background information necessary to navigate, understand, and complete each laboratory exercise contained herein. Additionally, the design of this lab guide is independent of an accompanying text book. Access to *A.D.A.M. Interactive Anatomy* (A.I.A.), www.interactiveanatomy.com, will allow the student to be completely immersed in a layer-by-layer virtual dissection experience. However, students without access to a computer, the Internet, or a companion text will still be afforded the opportunity to be successful, deepening their knowledge of important anatomical and physiological concepts presented in *A.D.A.M. Interactive Anatomy Online: Student Lab Activity Guide*.

WHAT IS NEW?

Navigation. New to this edition is the use of colorful icons to easily direct the student to corresponding images in A.I.A. While the crisp images in the text were chosen to reflect the most accurate content, accessing the actual images via A.I.A allows for further student exploration. When appropriate, icons alert students to alternate content areas within A.I.A, allowing them the opportunity to view additional images and deepen their understanding of the material. The following icons may be found throughout *A.D.A.M. Interactive Anatomy Online: Student Lab Activity Guide*:

Female (Eve) ♀ (view) (number); **Male (Adam)** ♂ (view) (number); **Dissectible Anatomy** DA;

Atlas Anatomy AA Surface of Tongue (Dorsal); **Clinical Illustrations** CI Dental Anatomy;

Clinical Animations ➔ Peristalsis, **3D Anatomy** 3D Skull.

Once the student has entered the appropriate A.I.A content area, he or she will be directed to the exact image by following the easy three-step navigation instructions provided in the text accompanying that image.

Four-color Design. The fourth edition of *A.D.A.M. Interactive Anatomy Online: Student Lab Activity Guide* has been beautifully redesigned using high-resolution, four-color images bringing out amazing detail and clarity of important anatomical structures. The high-resolution images allow the students to easily visualize these anatomical structures and give the instructors the diversity to choose from a multitude of impressive images for both instructional and testing purposes. To this end, the images have been created as "clean" images, that is, without the addition of "leader lines" pointing to specific structures. This allows for an unobstructed view of the appropriate structures and gives the instructor more flexibility when identifying organs as a whole or only those parts of the organs they find most meaningful.

Pedagogical Features. New pedagogical features included in the fourth edition allow for a uniform presentation throughout the lab guide. Each chapter begins with a set of *Learning Objectives*. The Learning Objectives clearly outline the types of information students should expect to learn while reading and completing the activities of the chapter. A *Chapter Overview* is included at the beginning of each chapter to introduce the student to the "big picture" regarding the design and function of the involved organ system. *Lab Activities* are designed to be succinct, complete, and to the appropriate level of students using this manual. A greater number of smaller, more manageable Lab Activities allows students to master one subject area before proceeding to the next. "Clean" images were purposely chosen for this manual for a twofold reason. First, they allow for greater instructor flexibility. When using A.I.A in a classroom setting, the instructor is better able to choose the best representation of the structures they are highlighting instead of being forced to use the exact location presented in the image. Secondly, a clean image allows for better student engagement. With preexisting leader lines and answer blanks, it is easier for students to rely on others, either fellow classmates or the guide itself, for locating anatomical structures. A clean image allows the instructors to tailor content to their classroom audience. Students are then expected to not only locate the structure visually, as with many other texts, but also draw their own lines (with instructor and peer guidance) and actually write in the name of the labeled structure. The extra step of self-labeling and writing the name of the appropriate structures helps to more thoroughly engage the students, encourages proper spelling, and helps them to better retain the learned material. Finally, each chapter ends with *Chapter Review Exercises*. Each set of Chapter Review Exercises contains a selection of matching, labeling, short answer, and essay-type questions. Each exercise has been created within the framework of the chapter content, providing the students with the materials necessary to complete the exercises without need for additional outside references. These exercises may be used as a self-study tool allowing students to monitor their own level of understanding or used by the instructor as a graded instrument to be handed in at the completion of each chapter.

Clinical Applications. Human anatomy and physiology challenges students to integrate inherently difficult concepts in a way that is manageable and understandable. *Clinical Applications* have been included in the fourth edition in an effort to make this difficult content more meaningful and applicable by introducing students to common pathologies, treatments, and lab tests routinely encountered in allied health. It is common for the introductory A&P student to ask "why do we need to know this?" or "what is going to be on the test?" The Clinical Applications will hopefully provide a little real-world excitement for the student and encourage them to engage in a mastery of the subject matter as they find out the real reason "they have to know this"... for the care of their future patients/clients.

User's Guide

This User's Guide shows you how to put the features of *A.D.A.M. Interactive Anatomy Online: Student Lab Activity Guide, Fourth Edition,* to work for you.

LEARNING OBJECTIVES

Each chapter begins with a list of Learning Objectives that clearly outline the types of information students should expect to learn while reading and completing the activities of the chapter.

LEARNING OBJECTIVES

Upon completion of this chapter, the student should be able to:

■ Describe the major functions of the muscular system
■ Describe common muscle origins and insertions as well as synergists and antagonists for major muscle groups
■ Provide examples of criteria used when naming muscles
■ Locate and identify the major muscles of the head and neck
■ Locate and identify the major muscles of the chest and back
■ Locate and identify the major muscles of the upper extremity
■ Locate and identify the major muscles of the lower extremity

Chapter Overview

Following the Learning Objectives, the Chapter Overview introduces the student to the "big picture" regarding the design and function of the involved organ system.

MUSCULAR SYSTEM OVERVIEW

Of the three types of muscle tissue in the body (skeletal, cardiac, and smooth), skeletal muscle is the only type to be under voluntary control. While all three muscle types can contract and produce movement, it is skeletal muscle that is primarily responsible for the movement of the body. Skeletal muscle allows for locomotion (walking) as well as smaller, more coordinated movements such as writing, driving, and even smiling. Some skeletal muscles are arranged in circular patterns around hollow passages (sphincters) controlling the movement of substances along those passages such as with urination and defecation. Skeletal muscles are continuously making small adjustments here and there to help us maintain our posture and hold our body position (so you do not fall out of your seat while reading this). As muscles use ATP for energy, they give off heat as a by-product of muscle contraction. This heat then helps us to maintain our normal body temperature. If you have ever experienced shivering, you know your muscles will contract involuntarily when you get cold in an attempt to help warm your body. Skeletal muscles can also help provide some protection. They have a limited ability to protect internal organs, such as those in the abdominal cavity. Also, while the action of many muscles is to cause movement at joints, they can also serve to stabilize and protect the joints. While a strain is damage to a muscle or tendon, a sprain is damage to a ligament that connects bone to bone. It is common practice to strengthen surrounding muscles after a sprain (of the knee, for example) in an attempt to stabilize the affected joint.

Lab Activities

Lab Activities encourage students to interact with A.I.A by providing step-by-step instructions for locating a specific image in the program. Then, drawing in lines and writing the labels for specific structures engages students, encourages proper spelling, and helps them to better retain the material.

LAB ACTIVITY 2.2

Muscles of the Trunk and Arm
The muscles of the trunk have a wide array of functions. Many of the muscles help to move the head and neck as well as the upper limb, including those that stabilize the scapulae. Since several muscles of the trunk cross the shoulder joint and act on the humerus, they will be considered in this section as well. The major, superficial muscle of the chest is the **pectoralis major**. The major muscle of the anterior arm, the **biceps brachii**, crosses both the shoulder and the elbow joints and allows for flexion of both joints. Antagonistic to the biceps brachii, the **triceps brachii** is the posterior arm counterpart. The **deltoid** muscle has anterior and posterior attachments to the shoulder girdle and is the main abductor of the arm. The **intercostal** muscles, along with the **pectoralis minor**, act on the ribs to aid respiration. The superficial, posterior muscles of the back are made up of the more superior **trapezius** and the inferior **latissimus dorsi** muscles. Deep posterior muscles help to support and move the vertebral column. While the abdominal muscles act on the vertebral column as well, they also offer some protection of the underlying viscera of the abdominal cavity.

Identify and label the superficial anterior muscles including the deltoid, pectoralis major, biceps brachii, and sternocleidomastoid in the figure below. The external oblique and the origin of the serratus anterior may also be seen here. To view the image in AIA, go to

DA ♂ A10 or DA ♀ A13

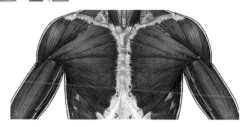

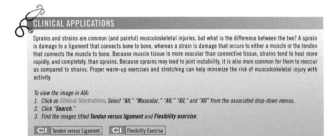

CLINICAL APPLICATIONS

Sprains and strains are common (and painful) musculoskeletal injuries, but what is the difference between the two? A sprain is damage to a ligament that connects bone to bone, whereas a strain is damage that occurs to either a muscle or the tendon that connects the muscle to bone. Because muscle tissue is more vascular than connective tissue, strains tend to heal more rapidly, and completely, than sprains. Because sprains may lead to joint instability, it is also more common for them to reoccur as compared to strains. Proper warm-up exercises and stretching can help minimize the risk of musculoskeletal injury with activity.

To view the image in AIA:
1. Click on Clinical Illustrations; Select "All," "Muscular," "All," "All," and "All" from the associated drop-down menus.
2. Click "Search."
3. Find the images titled Tendon versus ligament and Flexibility exercise.

CI Tendon versus Ligament   **CI** Flexibility Exercise

Clinical Applications

Throughout the chapters, Clinical Applications boxes help make chapter content more meaningful and applicable by introducing students to common pathologies, treatments, and lab tests routinely encountered in allied health.

MUSCULAR SYSTEM REVIEW EXERCISES

Matching

_____ **1.** Muscle named for orientation of fibers
_____ **2.** Muscle named for location
_____ **3.** Muscle named for number of origins
_____ **4.** Muscle named for shape
_____ **5.** Muscle named for its origin and insertion
_____ **6.** Muscle named for its size
_____ **7.** Muscle named for its action

a. depressor anguli oris
b. trapezius
c. rectus femoris
d. tibialis anterior
e. triceps brachii
f. coracobrachialis
g. gluteus minimus

Chapter Review Exercises

Each chapter ends with a Chapter Review Exercises section that contains a selection of matching, labeling, short answer, and essay-type questions. These questions may be used as a self-study tool allowing students to monitor their own level of understanding or used by the instructor as a graded instrument to be handed in at the completion of each chapter.

Instructor Resources

Online Instructor Resources include answer keys, an instructor's manual, and image bank.

Reviewers

Matthew Bruder
Professor
Department of Biological Sciences
DeVry University
Addison, Illinois

Susan Capasso, BA, MS, EdD
Dean Academic Services
Professor (Science)
St. Vincent's College
Bridgeport, Connecticut

Jim Cross, ND, BS
Anatomy/Physiology/Math Instructor
Feather River College
Quncy, California

Darrell Davies
Professor of Human Anatomy and Physiology
Kalamazoo Valley Community College
Kalamazoo, Michigan

Mark Jaffe, DPM, MHSA
Associate Professor
Division of Math, Science, and Technology
Nova Southeastern University
Fort Lauderdale-Davie, Florida

Jessica Kilham
Information & Education Services Librarian
Lyman Maynard Stowe Library
UCONN Health Center
Farmington, Connecticut

Will Kleinelp
Associate Professor
Department of Biology
Middlesex County College
Edison, New Jersey

Randy Taylor
Anatomy and Physiology Teacher
Science Department
McEachern High School
Powder Springs, Georgia

William R. Tobin
Assistant Professor
Department of Biology
Erie Community College–South Campus
Orchard Park, New York

Sara Sybesma Tolsma, PhD
Professor of Biology
Northwestern College
Orange City, Iowa

Acknowledgments

I have been so blessed to have the opportunity to create this fourth edition, and it is because of the support and confidence of many individuals that this final product has been created.

I would like to extend a sincere thank you to past members of the A.D.A.M. Education family, Maribel Brogden and Shannon McGuire, who had the confidence to welcome me into the world of online publishing and gave me the freedom to run with new ideas. A big thank you goes to Bridget Benware, current Sales Manager, Strategic Partnerships at A.D.A.M. Education, who kept my dream of writing alive by introducing me to the publishing team at Lippincott Williams & Wilkins/Wolters Kluwer Health. Thanks also to Jennifer Hickey at A.D.A.M. for managing the image files selected for use in this edition.

This fourth edition would not have been possible without the tremendous support and guidance of the talented, and patient, staff at Lippincott Williams & Wilkins. Special thanks to David Troy, Executive Editor, for taking a chance on a "newbie" and never wavering on his commitment to making this edition a superior product. This lab guide could have never been written without the exceptional skills and efforts of Amy Millholen, Senior Product Manager. Her tireless support, editing skills, and all-around approachability made my first experience as an author an enjoyable one. There are so many others behind the scenes at LWW who deserve recognition for their efforts in bringing this lab guide to life. The editing team, production team, and marketing team all did a stellar job of making my "vision" for this fourth edition tangible and assuring it was appropriate for the students who will benefit most from this effort.

I would like to offer my thanks to the countless students, patients, and colleagues over the years who have challenged me, taught me, encouraged me, and supported me in my quest to make the study of the human body a fun and welcoming experience. A special thank you goes to my colleague and friend, Wendy Rappazzo, for having the insight to use A.D.A.M. Interactive Anatomy in the HCC laboratory before I ever set foot on campus and for the selfless mentoring she has provided in the classroom.

While I knew it would be a challenge researching, gathering images, writing, and editing by the benchmarked deadlines, those efforts wouldn't have been possible without the unwavering support of my family. I would like to thank my parents, Bob and Linda Miller, for always believing in me and teaching me that it wasn't enough to get the job done—it had to be done right; and Dave and Judy Schaeffer, who would be proud of me even without this book. I have to thank my children, Dylan, Zachary, and Abigail, who had to endure quite a few boring days and weekends as dad was zoned out in front of the computer screen. I hope to be a source of pride and inspiration to you and can only hope that you find a vocation in life you will enjoy as much as I enjoy my role as an educator. I love you very much! Finally, I would like to express my sincerest thanks to my wife, Gay. I am so glad that I picked you! You made my rough days seem not-so-rough, made my good days better, endured my occasional moodiness, and settled for some lonely days and nights while my best efforts were directed into creating this lab guide. You offer unwavering support and encouragement, and you have continued to believe in me regardless of what has been on my plate. The creation of this fourth edition is so much more meaningful because I have the chance to share it with you.

Scott D. Schaeffer

Contents

About the Author v
A Note to Students vii
Preface ix
User's Guide xi
Reviewers xiii
Acknowledgments xv

Introduction   1

Chapter 1: Skeletal System   9

Chapter 2: Muscular System   33

Chapter 3: Nervous System   51

Chapter 4: Special Senses   71

Chapter 5: Endocrine System   87

Chapter 6: Cardiovascular System   103

Chapter 7: Lymphatic System   127

Chapter 8: Respiratory System   137

Chapter 9: Digestive System   147

Chapter 10: Urinary System   169

Chapter 11: Reproductive System   183

Introduction

Thank you for choosing *A.D.A.M. Interactive Anatomy Online: Student Lab Activity Guide* to help meet your educational needs. *A.D.A.M. Interactive Anatomy Online: Student Lab Activity Guide* is designed to accompany *A.D.A.M. Interactive Anatomy Online (AIA)* and is best utilized when access to www.interactiveanatomy.com is available. The following instructions are offered to help you navigate *AIA* while using this text. You will find that all of the images referenced in this text are available in *AIA* and may be accessed by following the instructions accompanying each image. Since one of the greatest strengths of *AIA* is the ability for "virtual dissection" using its vast image bank, each Lab Activity contained within provides critical background information to help you integrate the physiology associated with the structures identified within the *AIA* images.

A.D.A.M. Interactive Anatomy Online: Student Lab Activity Guide also contains several "Clinical Application" sections within each chapter. Each of these Clinical Applications highlights a common condition or pathology likely to be encountered in a typical health care setting. Where applicable, you will be directed to explore such *AIA* features as Clinical Images, Clinical Animations, or the Encyclopedia to reinforce the clinical application information presented in the *A.D.A.M. Interactive Anatomy Online: Student Lab Activity Guide*.

Chapter Review Exercises are found at the end of each chapter of the *Lab Activity Guide*. Instructors may opt to have you complete the Review Exercises to be collected and graded following the completion of each chapter or perhaps allow you to complete the exercises in the classroom setting, assessing your level of comprehension upon completion of the chapter lab activities. The Review Exercises include matching, labeling, fill-in-the-blank, and short answer/essay-type questions designed to reinforce the concepts presented in *A.D.A.M. Interactive Anatomy Online: Student Lab Activity Guide*.

INTRODUCTION TO *A.D.A.M. INTERACTIVE ANATOMY ONLINE*

A.D.A.M. Interactive Anatomy Online is a mainstay in anatomy education classes around the globe. This interactive learning system dramatically enhances the study of human anatomy and related topics with incredibly detailed graphics, precision accuracy, and advanced functionality. The newest edition is the best edition ever, with enhancements based on input from educators, authors, health professionals, and students worldwide. The result is the most innovative online anatomy reference and authoring system available. It's the most advanced curriculum development tool for instructors and a valuable lifelong anatomy resource for students.

LEARNING TO USE *A.D.A.M. INTERACTIVE ANATOMY ONLINE*

Open *AIA* by visiting www.interactiveanatomy.com and entering your username and password. This will take you to the Web site "homepage" where the list of resources is displayed along the left side of the screen.

Opening Anatomy Content

To open a dissectible anatomy view, an atlas anatomy image, a 3D anatomy model, a clinical illustration, or a clinical animation:

1. On the Resources screen, click the button for the type of content you want to open.

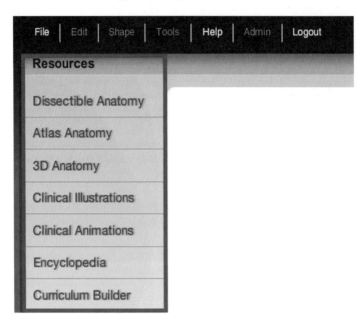

2. Choose the appropriate options for the content you would like to open. The Open dialog box displays the appropriate options for the content type.
3. To open multiple content types, first open one resource and then select "File" from the top menu bar and select "Open Resources." Next, select the additional resource you would like to open.
4. Click Open. *A.D.A.M. Interactive Anatomy* opens the selected content.

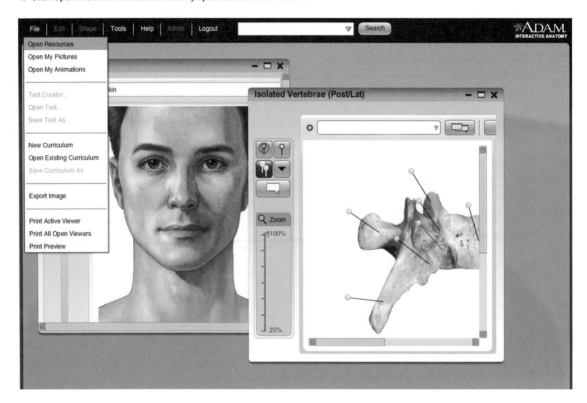

Dissectible Anatomy

Exercises using the Dissectible Anatomy images are indicated by the pink Dissectible Anatomy icon DA.
Upon selecting the Dissectible Anatomy resource within *AIA*, you have a choice of Gender and a choice of View
to access the appropriate image for each exercise.

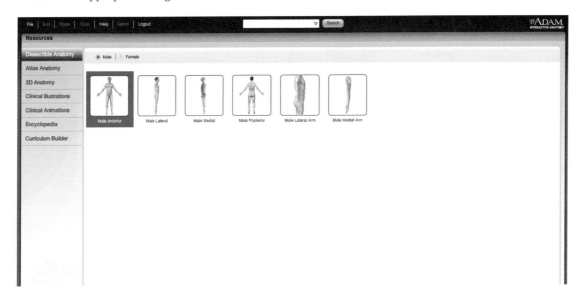

Many of the images used in this *Lab Guide* may be viewed in either the female or male gender, so both
options will made available when appropriate. The following icons have been included in the individual exercise
instructions to help you navigate to the exact images referenced in each exercise. Female images will be indicated by the female icon ♀, while male images will be indicated by the male icon ♂. Included next to each of
the gender icons is a letter indicating the appropriate view (A—anterior; P—posterior; M—medial; L—lateral)
and a number indicating the layer you will need to scroll down to using the depth bar found along the left side
of the screen.

As an example, try to find the following image in *AIA*. Begin by selecting Dissectible Anatomy DA from the
choices along the left side of the screen. Next select either ♀ A193 or ♂ A196 . Your computer screen should
now be displaying the following image:

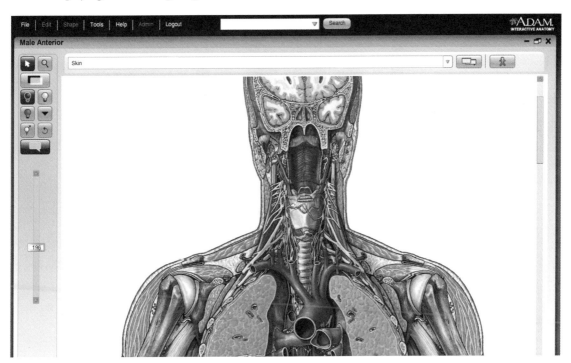

QUICK REFERENCE FOR WORKING WITH DISSECTIBLE ANATOMY

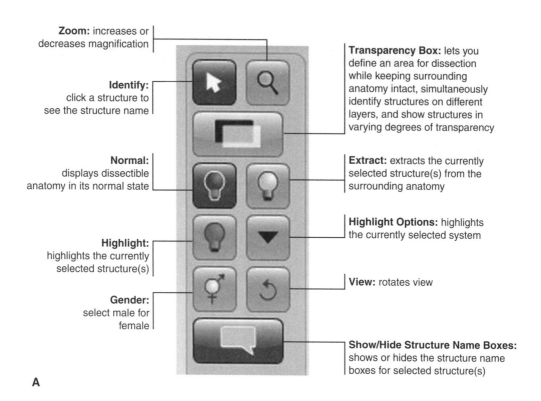

Zoom: increases or decreases magnification

Transparency Box: lets you define an area for dissection while keeping surrounding anatomy intact, simultaneously identify structures on different layers, and show structures in varying degrees of transparency

Identify: click a structure to see the structure name

Normal: displays dissectible anatomy in its normal state

Extract: extracts the currently selected structure(s) from the surrounding anatomy

Highlight Options: highlights the currently selected system

Highlight: highlights the currently selected structure(s)

View: rotates view

Gender: select male for female

Show/Hide Structure Name Boxes: shows or hides the structure name boxes for selected structure(s)

A

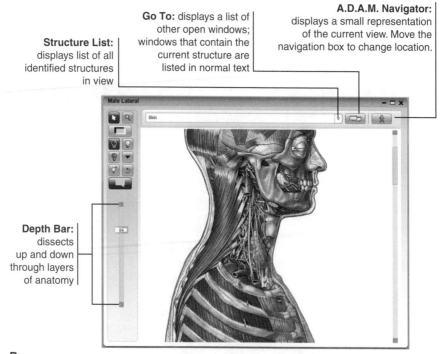

Structure List: displays list of all identified structures in view

Go To: displays a list of other open windows; windows that contain the current structure are listed in normal text

A.D.A.M. Navigator: displays a small representation of the current view. Move the navigation box to change location.

Depth Bar: dissects up and down through layers of anatomy

B

Atlas Anatomy

Exercises in the *Lab Guide* using the Atlas Anatomy images are indicated by the brown Atlas Anatomy icon **AA**. All Atlas Anatomy images are identified by a specific label that is included in the exercise directions as follows: **AA** Liver (Inf). You may view the entire library of Atlas Anatomy images from the **AA** screen, or you may narrow your search by using the image filters found along the top of the screen. You may narrow your search by selecting the appropriate **Body Region** and **Body System** that corresponds to the exercise, as well as the **View Orientation**. Additionally, the displayed images may be categorized by **Image Type** including **Illustration**, **Cadaver Photograph**, and **Radiograph** images, depending on the image referenced in the corresponding *Lab Guide* exercise.

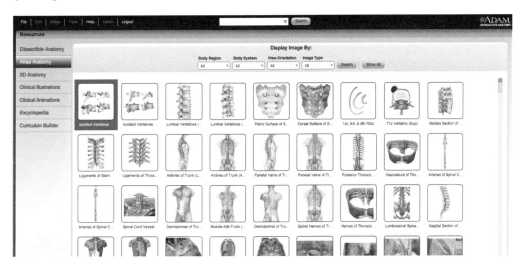

As an example, try to find the following image in *AIA*: **AA** Liver (Inf). Begin by selecting Atlas Anatomy **AA** from the choices along the left side of the screen. Next, either simply scroll down until you find the **Liver (Inf)** image from the selections on your screen, or filter the search by **Body Region** (Abdomen), **Body System** (Digestive), and **Image Type** (Illustration), and then click on "Search." This method will reduce the number of images displayed on your screen and make it easier to locate the desired image quickly.

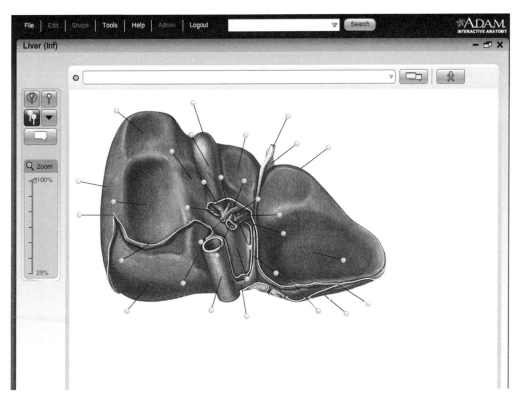

QUICK REFERENCE FOR WORKING WITH ATLAS ANATOMY

Hide Pins:
hides all structure pins
for the current image

Show Selected Pins:
displays only the pins
for the selected structures

Show All Pins In System(S):
displays all pins for
a selected
system

Select System:
displays all pins for
the selected system

Zoom:
Changes the zoom
level of the image

Show/Hide Structure Name Boxes:
shows or hides
the structure name
boxes for selected pin(s)

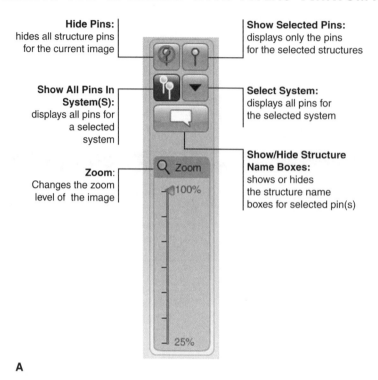

A

Structure List:
displays list of all
identified structures
in view

Go To:
displays a list of other
open windows; windows
that contain the current
structure are listed in
normal text

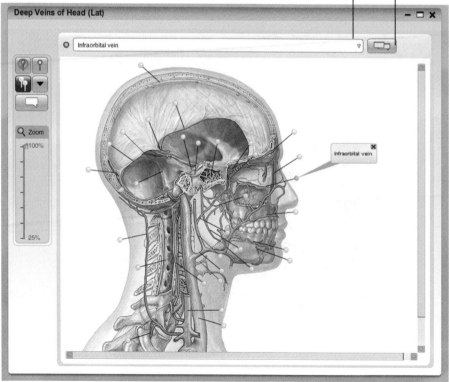

Deep Veins of Head (Lat)

Infraorbital vein

Infraorbital vein

B

Clinical Illustrations and Clinical Animations

In several exercises found in this *Lab Guide*, "Clinical Applications" are included to highlight common pathological conditions. These exercises include references to Clinical Illustrations and/or Clinical Animations found within the *AIA* program. Clinical Animations are indicated with this orange icon ➔. All Clinical Illustration images and Clinical Animations are identified by a specific label that is included in the Clinical Applications box in the same manner described above in the instructions for Atlas Anatomy. Also, in a similar fashion, both Clinical Illustrations and Clinical Animations may be filtered with the drop-down menus at the top of the screen to minimize the number of images displayed on your screen.

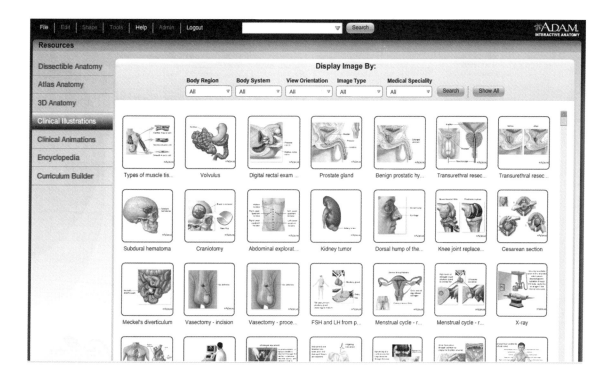

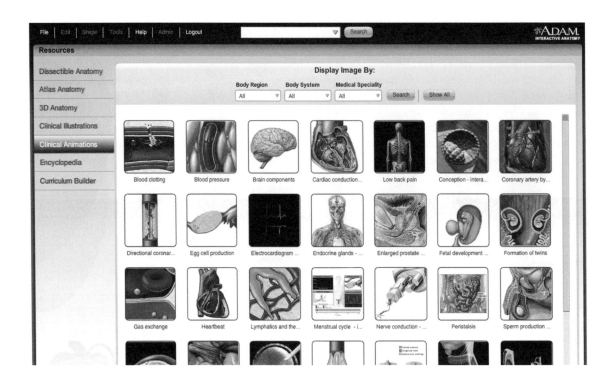

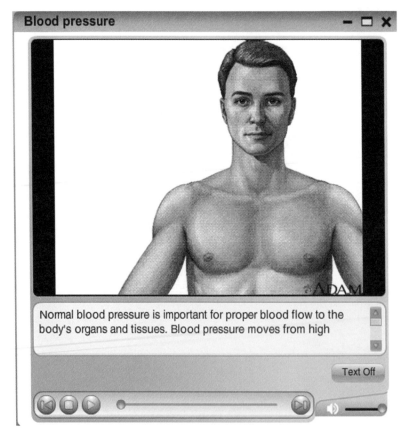

Skeletal System

LEARNING OBJECTIVES

Upon completion of this chapter, the student should be able to:

- Locate and identify the bones (and their features) of the axial skeleton

- Locate and identify the bones (and their features) of the appendicular skeleton

- Identify important internal and external features of the skull, including: surface features, sutures, foramina, sinuses, bones of the orbit, and fontanelles (in the fetal skull)

- Identify the primary and secondary curvatures of the spine and describe the vertebrae that contribute to the distinct regions of the spinal column

- Identify the regions of the sternum and distinguish between the different classifications of ribs

- Locate the bones of the pectoral girdle and upper extremity and identify their major surface markings

- Locate the bones of the pelvic girdle and lower extremity and identify their major surface markings

- Describe some differences between the female and male bony pelvis

- Be familiar with some of the more common pathological conditions of the skeletal system

SKELETAL SYSTEM OVERVIEW

The **skeletal system** is made up of 206 bones, cartilages, and ligamentous tissues that serve to provide support to the body and protect internal soft organs as well as provide attachments for skeletal muscles that are used to move the body. Additionally, the skeleton serves as a storage site for lipids and minerals such as calcium and phosphorus and as the site for hematopoiesis (blood cell production).

The skeleton is divided into two primary divisions: the **axial skeleton** (including the skull, vertebral column, and rib cage) and the **appendicular skeleton** (including the shoulder and pelvic girdles as well as the upper and lower extremities). Upon examination of the skeleton, it will be noticed that the bones are not smooth, but rather, they have various bumps, ridges, and openings that serve as sites of muscle attachment, articulations with other bones, and as passageways for blood vessels and nerves. Common names for bony projections that serve as attachment sites for tendons and ligaments include **tubercles, tuberosities, trochanters, crests, lines, spines,** and **rami (ramus)**. Common names for projections that help form articulations include **heads, processes, facets,** and **condyles**. Common names for openings or spaces in bones include **fissures, grooves, foramina (foramen), fossas, meatuses,** and **sinuses**. Familiarity with these terms will come in handy when identifying common features of the human skeleton in the laboratory setting.

SKULL OVERVIEW

The skull is composed of **8 cranial bones** that make up the **cranium** that encases and protects the brain and **14 facial bones** that serve as the basis for attachment for the muscles of facial expression. The cranial bones include the paired **parietal** and **temporal** bones as well as the single **frontal, occipital, sphenoid,** and **ethmoid** bones. The facial bones include the paired **maxilla, zygomatic, palatine, nasal, lacrimal,** and **inferior nasal conchae** in addition to the singular **mandible** and **vomer** bones.

*For a unique interactive experience, click on the 3D Anatomy icon and then select **3D Skull**.*

From there you are able to manipulate a three-dimensional skull by rotating it, moving it, zooming in and out, and even experience cutaway views.

 LAB ACTIVITY 1.1

Anterior View of the Skull

From this view of the skull, the **zygomatic**, **temporal**, **nasal**, **lacrimal**, **inferior nasal conchae**, and **parietal** bones are evident. The **frontal** bone with the **supraorbital margin** and **supraorbital foramen** (notch in some individuals) makes up the superior border of the orbit. In all, seven bones of the skull contribute to the orbit. *To view a close-up of the orbit in its entirety, click on* **AA** Walls of Orbit (Ant) . The **perpendicular plate** and **middle nasal conchae** of the **ethmoid** bone can be seen within the nasal cavity. The **vomer** (along with the perpendicular plate of the ethmoid bone) comprises the **nasal septum**. *To view the nasal septum in its entirety, click on* **DA** ♂ A49 *or* **DA** ♀ A49 *as well as* **DA** ♂ L209 *or* **DA** ♀ L210 . The **maxilla** (upper jaw) with the **infraorbital foramen** and the **ramus** and **body** of the **mandible** (lower jaw) with the **mental foramina** are easily seen from the anterior.

Identify and label the bones of the skull and their common markings visible from the anterior view in the following figure.

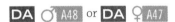

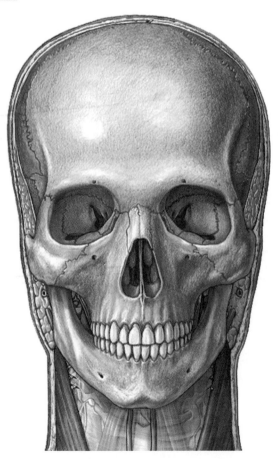

LAB ACTIVITY 1.2

Lateral View of the Skull

From the lateral view of the skull, the **frontal**, **parietal**, **nasal**, and **lacrimal** bones may be seen. At the anterior aspect of this view, the **alveolar processes** of the **maxilla** are seen, while at the inferior aspect the **occipital condyles** may be visualized. The **greater wing** of the **sphenoid** bone can be seen articulating with the **squamous** part of the **temporal** bone. The temporal bone has several visible features in this view. The **mastoid process** may be found just inferior and posterior to the **external acoustic meatus**. The **zygomatic arch** is made from the union of the **zygomatic process** of the temporal bone and the **temporal process** of the **zygomatic** bone. The **body**, **ramus**, and **angle** of the **mandible** along with the **condylar process** (contributing to the **temporal mandibular joint**) and **coronoid process** may be visualized. Finally, three sutures are visible from the lateral aspect of the skull. The **frontal suture** is made from the union of the frontal bone and parietal bones; the **squamosal suture** is between the parietal and temporal bones; and the **lambdoid suture** is the connection between the occipital bones and the two parietal bones.

Identify and label the bones of the skull and their common markings visible from the lateral view in the following figure.

AA Skull (Lat) 1

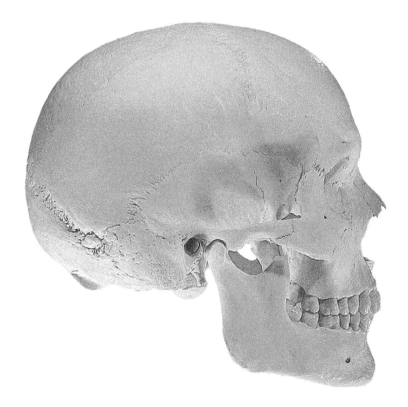

To view comparable landmarks of the lateral skull, go to **DA** ♂ L118 *or* **DA** ♀ L118 . The **hyoid bone** is not considered a bone of the skull but will be included here since it is visible in this view. The hyoid bone is the only bone in the human skeleton that does not articulate with another bone. It serves as a point of attachment for several muscles of the tongue and larynx.

LAB ACTIVITY 1.3

Posterior View of the Skull

The posterior view of the skull has but a few key landmarks worth noting. The **sagittal suture** is seen joining the left and right **parietal** bones. The **lambdoid suture** between the **occipital** bone and **parietal** bones may be seen also. Other features of the occipital bone include the **external occipital protuberance** (EOP, inion) and the **superior** and **inferior nuchal lines**. The **mastoid process** of the **temporal** bone can also be seen from the posterior view.

Identify and label the bones of the skull and their common markings visible from the posterior view in the following figure.

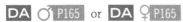

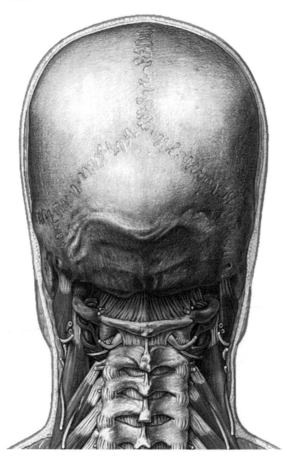

LAB ACTIVITY 1.4

Inferior View of the Skull

The inferior aspect of the skull can be very intimidating with the abundance of projections, depressions, and openings, but with some practice (and patience), the following bones and markings may be identified. The **hard palate** is seen as the two **palatine processes** of the maxillae join with the two **horizontal plates** of the palatine bones. The rather large **incisive fossa** may be found at the most anterior aspect. Posterior to the palatine bones and in the midline is the **vomer**. Several foramina may be visualized in the **sphenoid** bone for the passing of cranial nerves. They include the **foramen ovale** and **foramen spinosum** in addition to the **foramen lacerum** that shares a border with the temporal bone. Other openings in the temporal bone include the **carotid canal** and the **stylomastoid foramen** that is nestled between the **mastoid process** and **styloid process**. The **mandibular fossa** receives the **head** (**condylar process**) of the mandible to form the temporomandibular joint (TMJ). Anterolateral to the mandibular fossa, the **zygomatic process** may be seen from below. The largest opening in the base of the skull is the **foramen magnum** of the occipital bone, located medially to the paired **occipital condyles**. The **condylar canals** may be found just posterior to the condyles. Finally, the **external occipital crest** is visualized from this angle along with the **superior** and **inferior nuchal lines**.

Identify and label the bones of the skull and their common markings visible from the inferior view in the following figure.

AA Skull (Inf)

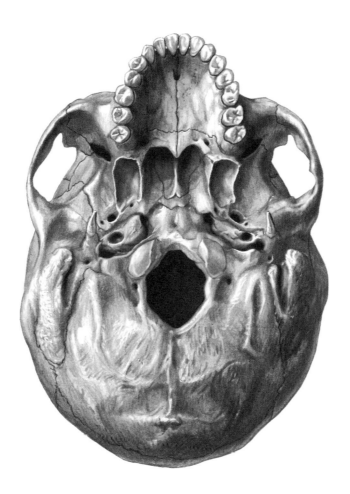

LAB ACTIVITY 1.5

Internal View of the Cranial Cavities

While viewing the interior aspect of the skull floor, three distinct regions may be visualized. The **anterior cranial fossa** encompasses the frontal and ethmoid bones; the **middle cranial fossa** is found between the lesser wings of the sphenoid bone and the petrous portion of the temporal bone; and the **posterior cranial fossa** sets upon the occipital bone. In the anterior cranial fossa, two features of the ethmoid bone are visualized. The raised **crista galli** serves as an attachment point for the dura mater, while the hole-riddled **cribriform plate** allows for olfactory nerve fibers to pass from the nasal mucosa to the brain. *To view the olfactory nerve's relationship to the ethmoid bone, click on* **AA** Olfactory Nerve in Nasal Cavity . The **sella turcica** of the sphenoid bone may be seen in the midline of the skull floor, situated between the **anterior** and **posterior clinoid processes**. The **hypophyseal fossa** is the depression within the sella turcica where the pituitary gland (hypophysis cerebri) is housed. Several openings in the skull floor can be visualized from the internal view. From anterior to posterior within the sphenoid bone are the **optic canal**, **superior orbital fissure**, **foramen rotundum**, **foramen ovale**, and the **foramen spinosum**. The large **foramen magnum** and smaller, paired **hypoglossal canals** may be seen within the occipital bone. Finally, within the temporal bone is found the **internal acoustic meatus,** while two other openings, the **foramen lacerum** and the **jugular foramen,** may be seen at its border.

Identify and label the bones of the skull and their common markings visible from the internal view in the following figure.

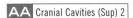

AA Cranial Cavities (Sup) 2

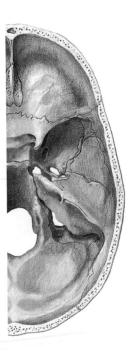

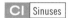

Paranasal Sinuses

Paranasal sinuses are mucosa-lined cavities within the skull that serve to lighten the skull, warm and humidify inspired air, and serve as resonance chambers for speech. The four skull bones that house the paranasal sinuses are the **frontal**, **maxillary**, **ethmoid,** and **sphenoid** bones.

Identify and label the bones of the skull that house paranasal sinuses in the following figure.

CI Sinuses

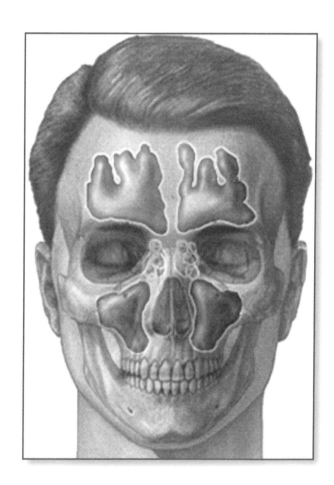

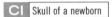 **LAB ACTIVITY 1.7**

The Fetal Skull

As with the rest of the skeleton, the bones of the fetal skull are incompletely formed at birth. This nonunion of the skull bones allows the bones to shift (or mold) slightly to allow for easier passage through the birth canal. Click on **CI** Fetal Head Molding to visualize this process. Six distinct fontanelles, or "soft spots," may be visualized at the junction of several cranial bones. The largest of these is the **anterior fontanelle** where the frontal (coronal) suture will eventually be found. Also in the midline can be found the **posterior fontanelle** where the lamboid suture will later be found. There are also two paired fontanelles—the **sphenoid (anterolateral)** and the **mastoid (posterolateral)** fontanelles. As the skull matures, the fontanelles should completely disappear by approximately 22 to 24 months of age.

Identify and label the fontanelles in the fetal skull in the following figure.

CI Skull of a newborn

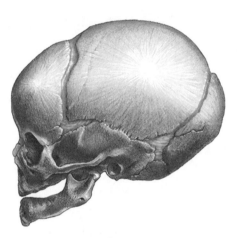

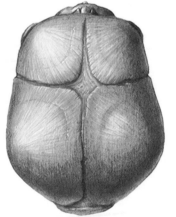

LAB ACTIVITY 1.8

The Vertebral Column

The vertebral (or spinal) column consists of 24 individual segments and 2 fused bones. There are **7 cervical**, **12 thoracic**, and **5 lumbar** vertebrae, all of which (except for C1/C2) are separated from each other by a fibrocartilage intervertebral disc (IVD). Five segments fuse together to give us a **sacrum**, while four segments fuse together to give us a **coccyx** (or tail bone). The **atlas (C1)** is unique in that it does not have a body but, instead, has an **anterior** and a **posterior arch**. The **axis (C2)** has a unique feature, the **dens** or **odontoid process**, which serves as a pivot point for the atlas to rotate (as in turning your head from side to side). All seven cervical vertebrae have a **transverse foramen** that allows for the passage of the vertebral artery. Each of the 12 thoracic vertebrae attaches to a corresponding rib and has **costal facets** (or demifacets) on the body for the attachment of the rib head and transverse costal facets for the attachment of the rib tubercle. The lumbar vertebrae are the thickest of all levels as they support the bulk of the axial stress of the body. The sacrum is unique in that the five segments of the fused sacrum are usually identifiable with the remnants of the IVDs seen as **transverse ridges**. The **anterior** and **posterior sacral foramina** allow for the exit of spinal nerves from the sacrum. Laterally are the wing-like **alae** that articulate with either side of the os coxae (pelvic bones) forming the **sacroiliac joints**. Posteriorly may be found the **median sacral crest** that is the remnant of the spinous processes of the sacral segments. The inferior aspect of the sacrum articulates with the **coccyx**, or tail bone.

With the exception of C1 and C2, the other 22 vertebrae all have similar "typical" features. The **body** (centrum) is the thickest part of the vertebra that attaches to the IVD. Extending posteriorly from the body are the paired **pedicles**. Paired **transverse processes** project laterally while a single **spinous process** projects posteriorly. Between the transverse and spinous processes is where the **laminae** are found. The **vertebral** (or spinal) **foramen** is the large opening in the neural arch for the passage of the spinal cord. Projecting upward from the neural arch are paired **superior articulating processes** (with an articulating facet), while the **inferior articulating process** are found in the opposite direction (also with an articulating facet).

Identify and label the spinal levels and typical features of the vertebrae in the following figures.

CI Skeletal Spine

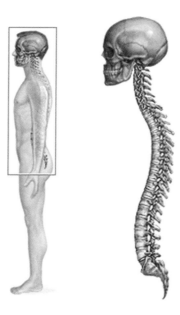

AA | Isolated Vertebrae (Ant/Lat)

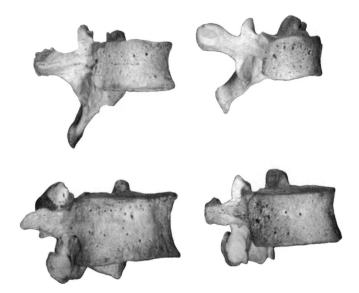

CLINICAL APPLICATIONS

The fetal spine is "C-shaped" in utero with a convex curvature to the posterior (kyphotic). Spinal curves that are kyphotic in nature are referred to as primary curves since they are present at birth. As the infant begins to crawl and lift the head, a secondary curve develops in the cervical spine (lordosis). Later, as the child moves from crawling to an upright posture, another secondary curvature develops in the lumbar spine. Three abnormal curvatures of the spine may develop as a result of trauma, degeneration, or abnormal muscle tone. A lateral curvature of the spine is known as scoliosis. A hyperkyphotic curvature of the thoracic spine is commonly known as a "hunchback," whereas a hyperlordosis of the lumbar spine is referred to as a "swayback."

To view some images of spinal curvatures in AIA:
1. *Click on Clinical Illustrations; Select **Skeletal**, **All**, **All**, **All**, and **All** from the drop-down menus.*
2. *Click "**Search**."*
3. *Find the images titled **Spinal Curves**, **Scoliosis**, **Signs of Scoliosis**, **Osteoporosis of the Spine**, and **Lordosis** to view the variations in spinal curvatures.*

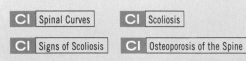

CI	Spinal Curves	**CI**	Scoliosis
CI	Signs of Scoliosis	**CI**	Osteoporosis of the Spine
CI	Lordosis

It is estimated that over 80% of the adult population will experience low back pain (LBP) at some point in their lives. Treatments for LBP may be as varied as the causes. While some treatments may be as simple as rest and stretching/strengthening exercises, other cases may require chiropractic, physical therapy, medication, or even surgery. Go to ➡ | Low Back Pain | to view an animation on LBP.

To view some images of intervertebral disc lesions in AIA:
1. *Click on Clinical Illustrations; Select "**Skeletal**," "**All**," "**All**," "**All**," and "**All**" from the drop-down menus.*
2. *Click "**Search**."*
3. *Find the images titled **Herniated Lumbar Disc**, **Herniated Nucleus Pulposus**, **Spinal Stenosis**, **Laminectomy—L4**, and **Lumbar Discectomy**, to view some causes and surgical treatments for LBP.*

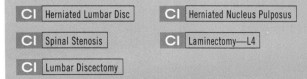

CI	Herniated Lumbar Disc	**CI**	Herniated Nucleus Pulposus
CI	Spinal Stenosis	**CI**	Laminectomy—L4
CI	Lumbar Discectomy

LAB ACTIVITY 1.9

The Sternum and Ribs

The **sternum**, or breastbone, is made from the union of three distinct bones. The most superior of these bones is the **manubrium**, with the **jugular notch** on its superior border. Laterally, the manubrium will articulate with the clavicle at the sternoclavicular joint. The largest section of the sternum is the **body** (gladiolus). The most inferior section is referred to as the **xiphoid process**.

Twelve pairs of ribs make up the thoracic cage. Ribs 1 to 7 are known as **true ribs** (vertebrosternal) and have individual cartilage attachments to the sternum. Ribs 8 to 12 are classified as **false ribs** and be further subdivided based on their articulations. Ribs 8 to 10 share a common cartilage attachment and are known as **vertebro-chondral ribs,** whereas ribs 11 and 12 have no anterior attachment and are classified as **floating** or **vertebral ribs**. The **head**, **neck**, **tubercle**, **angle**, and **body** of the ribs may be seen by clicking on AA 1st, 3rd, & 8th ribs .

Identify and label the regions of the sternum as well as the ribs in the following figure.

  A156 or A156

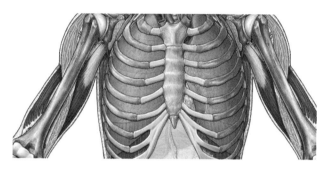

Try to compare as many features as you can identify from the illustration above to the Cadaver Photograph in the following image.

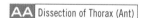 Dissection of Thorax (Ant)

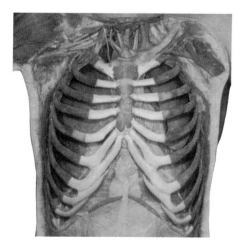

LAB ACTIVITY 1.10

The Pectoral (Shoulder) Girdle

The pectoral, or shoulder, girdle consists of two bones that connect the upper extremity to the axial skeleton—the **clavicle** (collarbone) and the **scapula** (shoulder blade). The **clavicle** is flat and S-shaped and articulates medially with the manubrium at the sternoclavicular joint and laterally with the scapula at the acromioclavicular joint. The **scapula** is a triangular-shaped bone with the lateral-most angle articulating with the humerus at the shallow **glenoid fossa**. The medial border faces the vertebral column whereas the lateral border faces the axilla (armpit). The **suprascapular notch** is visible along the superior border. The ventral aspect of the scapula rests against the rib cage and contains the **subscapular fossa**. A prominent ventral projection that serves as a muscular attachment is the **coracoid process**. The dorsal aspect of the scapula has a prominent ridge (**spine of the scapula**) that separates the **supraspinous fossa** from the **infraspinous fossa**. The spine of the scapula terminates laterally in a prominent projection called the **acromion process**, which articulates with the clavicle.

The Arm

The **humerus** is the single bone of the arm. Proximally, there are three prominent projections. The large, rounded **head** articulates medially with the scapula. The **greater tubercle** can be found laterally, while the **lesser tubercle** is found slightly medial and inferior. Between the tubercles is the **intertubercular groove** that houses the tendon of the long head of the biceps brachii. The **anatomical neck** is found encircling the head, while the surgical neck, a common site of fracture, is found around the proximal metaphysis of the humerus. The **deltoid tuberosity** is a broad, roughened region on the lateral aspect of the shaft where the deltoid muscle has its insertion. Distally, the humeral condyles are known as the medial **trochlea** that articulates with the ulna and the lateral **capitulum** that articulates with the radius. Just proximally and wide to the condyles are the two **epicondyles**. The shallow **coronoid fossa** on the anterior surface and the deeper **olecranon fossa** posteriorly allow room for the corresponding ulnar processes during flexion and extension of the elbow joint.

Identify and label the bones of the pectoral girdle and arm, along with their features, in the following figures.

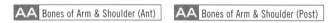

| **AA** Bones of Arm & Shoulder (Ant) | **AA** Bones of Arm & Shoulder (Post) |

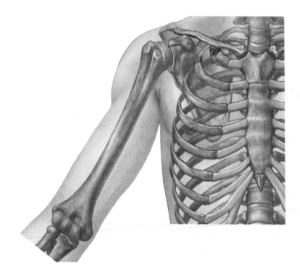
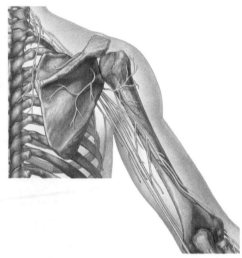

LAB ACTIVITY 1.11

The Forearm

The forearm is formed by two parallel bones—the **radius** laterally and the **ulna** medially. The **head** of the radius articulates proximally with the **capitulum** of the humerus. Just distal and medial to the head is the **radial tuberosity**, which serves as the insertion for the biceps brachii muscle. The **styloid process** may be seen as the most distal projection of the radius. The proximal ulna has the large **olecranon process** to the posterior and the smaller **coronoid process** to the anterior. The head of the ulna is at the distal end of the bone and has the small **styloid process** projecting of its medial aspect.

The Hand

The hand is made up of 27 bones that are divided into three distinct groups: the carpals (wrist), metacarpals, and phalanges (fingers). The eight **carpals** are divided into a proximal row (from lateral to medial—scaphoid, lunate, triquetral, pisiform) and a distal row (from lateral to medial—trapezium, trapezoid, capitate, hamate). The five **metacarpals** are found within the palm of the hand and are numbered 1 to 5 beginning laterally with the thumb (**pollex**). Digits 2 to 5 have three **phalanges** each (proximal, middle, distal) while the thumb only has two (proximal and distal).

Identify and label the bones of forearm and hand, along with their features, in the following figures.

| AA | Bones of Forearm & Hand (Ant) | | AA | Bones of Forearm & Hand (Post) |

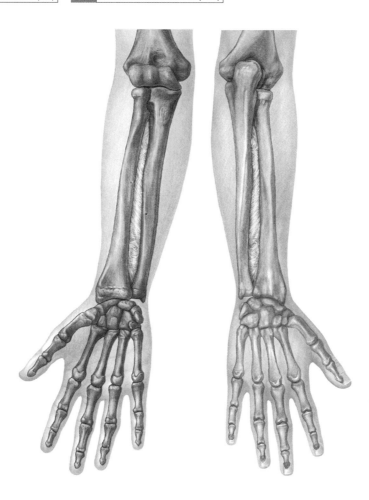

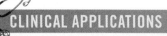

CLINICAL APPLICATIONS

Arthritis is a very general term that simply refers to the inflammation of a joint. Two of the most common forms of arthritis seen clinically are **osteoarthritis (OA)** and **rheumatoid arthritis (RA)**. Osteoarthritis is often referred to as the *"wear and tear"* form of arthritis and usually results from overuse, repetitive trauma, and aging. The symptoms of OA generally get worse over time but can be treated with conservative methods such as chiropractic and physical therapy to slow the progression of the disease as well as the use of some over-the-counter medications to help alleviate discomfort. OA is also known as *degenerative joint disease (DJD)*. X-ray changes may show bone wearing down at the ends of the bone, bone spur formation (osteophytes), and a decrease in joint space. Symptoms usually appear in middle age and include pain and stiffness in the joint with a limited range of motion. **Rheumatoid arthritis** is an autoimmune disease where the immune system of the individual attacks healthy joint tissues. RA can occur at any age but is more common in middle age and tends to affect women more than men. RA tends to affect the body bilaterally, with the most affected joints including the fingers, wrist, knees, feet, and ankles. Over time, joints may lose their range of motion and even become deformed. While OA symptoms are restricted to the joint, RA can affect other tissues as well such as the lungs, heart, and blood vessels. Treatment of RA usually includes medications to prevent inflammation and suppress immune function along with therapeutic treatment to reduce swelling and discomfort. Surgical correction is sometimes necessary to treat joint deformation and immobilization.

To view some images of osteoarthritis and rheumatoid arthritis in AIA:
1. *Click on Clinical Illustrations; Select "All," "Skeletal," "All," "All," and "Orthopedics" from the associated drop-down menus.*
2. *Click "Search."*
3. *Find the corresponding images.*

 LAB ACTIVITY 1.12

The Pelvic Girdle

The pelvic girdle is formed by the two hip bones (ossa coxae or pelvic bones). Posteriorly, the pelvic bones are joined to the sacrum at the sacroiliac joint, and anteriorly, they connect at the fibrocartilage pubic symphysis. Each **os coxae** is actually formed by the union of three separate bones—the ilium, ischium, and pubis. The **ilium** has the iliac crest at the most superior aspect of the bone. Anteriorly, the **iliac crest** ends at the **anterior superior iliac spine**, while posteriorly it ends at the **posterior superior iliac spine**. Just below each superior iliac spine can be found a corresponding **inferior iliac spine**. The **ischium** is known as the "butt" bone, and the brunt of the body weight rests on the **ischial tuberosity** when in the seated position. The **ischial spine** projects posteriorly and separates the superior **greater sciatic notch** from the inferior **lesser sciatic notch**. The **ramus** of the ischium connects to the **inferior pubic ramus** anteriorly. Then, with the addition of the **superior pubic ramus**, the large **obturator foramen** is formed. The two pubic bones are joined anteriorly at the **pubic symphysis**. Laterally, the individual bones of the os coxae unite at the **acetabulum**, or hip socket, which receives the head of the femur to make the hip joint.

Identify and label the bones of pelvic girdle, along with their features, in the following figures.

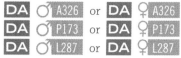

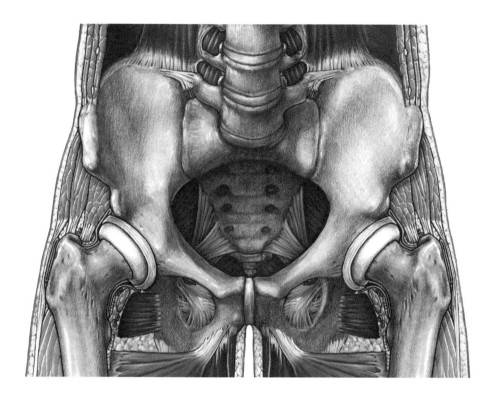

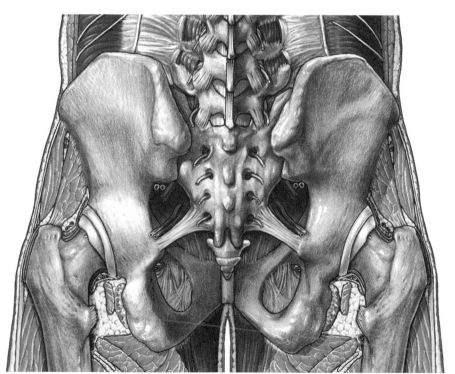

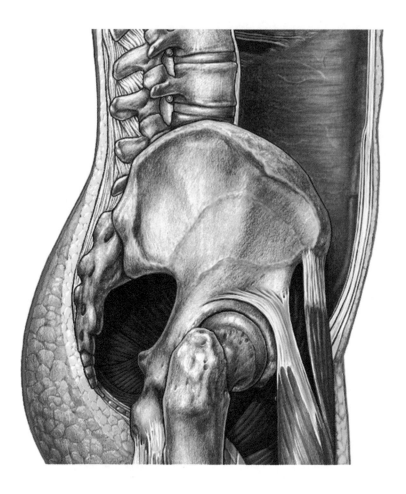

CLINICAL APPLICATIONS

Joint replacement surgeries are becoming increasingly popular as the numbers of the geriatric population continue to rise. Two of the most commonly replaced joints are the weight-bearing joints of the lower extremity, the hip joint and knee joint. You have probably heard someone say that they had fallen and broken their hip. In all likelihood, though, it was the opposite—they broke their hip, which caused them to fall. To make matters more confusing, it is not their "hip" that has broken at all but rather the neck of their femur. Osteoporosis, arthritis, injury, and even a history of certain medications are a few reasons that may lead to the need for a total joint replacement.

To view some images of knee and hip joint replacement surgeries in AIA:
1. *Click on "Clinical Illustrations"; select "**Lower Limb**," "**Skeletal**," "**All**," "**All**," and "**Orthopedics**" from the associated drop-down menus.*
2. *Click "**Search**."*
3. *Find the corresponding images.*

LAB ACTIVITY 1.13

The Thigh

The **femur**, the largest and heaviest bone in the body, is the single bone of the thigh. Its **head** articulates proximally with the acetabulum as it forms a deep, stable ball-and-socket type joint. At the inferior aspect of the femoral **neck** may be found two trochanters. The larger, **greater trochanter** is found laterally while the smaller **lesser trochanter** is found medially and slightly inferior. The more prominent **intertrochanteric crest** connects the two posteriorly while the **intertrochanteric line** connects them anteriorly. The **linea aspera** is a raised ridge that runs down the posterior aspect of the femoral shaft and serves as an attachment point for several muscles of the thigh. The distal end of the femur articulates with the tibia at the **medial** and **lateral condyles**. The **patellar surface** is found between the condyles on the anterior aspect and serves as an articulation site for the patella (kneecap). The medial and lateral **epicondyles** are found just above their respective condyles. On the medial aspect of the distal femur is an additional projection, the **adductor tubercle**, an insertion point for the powerful adductor muscles of the thigh.

Identify and label the features of the femur, along with the proximal and distal articulating bones, in the following figures.

| AA | Bones of Lower Limb (Ant) | | AA | Bones of Lower Limb (Post) |

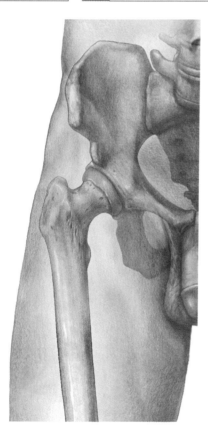
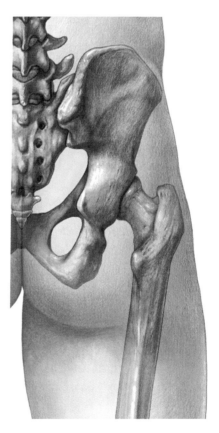

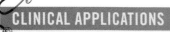

CLINICAL APPLICATIONS

Advances in surgical techniques have allowed for minimally invasive joint surgery, known as **arthroscopic surgery**, which generally allows patients to return home the same day the procedure is performed. With arthroscopic surgery, several buttonhole-sized incisions are made in the skin for the insertion of an *arthroscope* (instrument to view the joint space) and various arthroscopic surgical instruments. Arthroscopic examination not only allows the physician to make a more definitive diagnosis of joint injury and disease but it also allows for a prompt surgical correction when indicated.

To view some images of arthroscopy in AIA:
1. Click on Clinical Illustrations; Select "All," "Skeletal," "All," "All," and "Orthopedics" from the associated drop-down menus.
2. Click "Search."
3. Find the corresponding images.

 LAB ACTIVITY 1.14

The Leg

The leg is formed by two parallel bones—the larger, medial tibia (shin bone) and the thin, lateral fibula. The **tibia** is the weight-bearing bone of the leg and has the **medial** and **lateral condyles** proximally to articulate with the corresponding condyles of the femur at the knee joint. Between the tibial condyles is the raised **intercondylar eminence**. The **tibial tuberosity** is the prominent bump on the anterior aspect of the tibia that serves as the insertion point of the patellar ligament. Distally, the tibia articulates with the talus at the tibiotalar (ankle) joint. The rounded knob on the medial aspect is the **medial malleolus** while the **fibular notch** (on the lateral aspect) receives the **lateral malleolus** of the **fibula**. The proximal end of the fibula, the **head**, does not contribute to the knee joint but instead articulates with the lateral condyle of the tibia.

CLINICAL APPLICATIONS

Irritation of the tibial tuberosity in adolescents causes a condition of pain and inflammation known as Osgood-Schlatter disease.
1. Click on Clinical Illustrations; Select "Skeletal," "All," "All," "All," and "All" from the drop-down menus.
2. Click "Search."
*3. Find the images titled **Leg Pain (Osgood-Schlatter)**.*

CI   Leg Pain (Osgood-Schlatter)

Identify and label the bones of the leg, along with their features, in the figure below.

AA Bones of Leg & Foot (Ant)

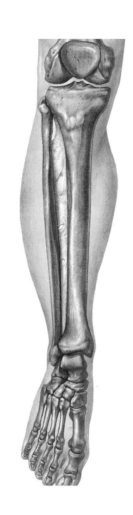

LAB ACTIVITY 1.15

The Foot

The foot is made of up 26 bones that are divided into three distinct groups: the tarsals (ankle), metatarsals, and phalanges (toes). The seven **tarsals** of the ankle are the talus (articulates with the tibia), calcaneus (heel bone), navicular, the cuneiforms (medial, intermediate, lateral), and the cuboid. The five **metatarsals** form the sole of the foot and are numbered 1 to 5 beginning medially with the great toe (**hallux**). Digits 2 to 5 have three **phalanges** each (proximal, middle, distal) while the hallux only has two (proximal and distal).

Identify and label the bones of foot and ankle in the following figure.

AA Bones of Foot (Dorsal)

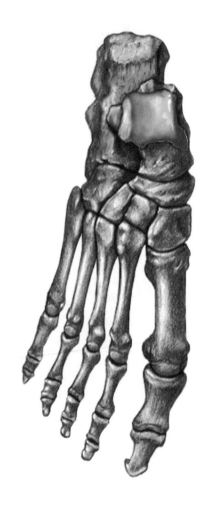

SKELETAL SYSTEM REVIEW EXERCISES

Matching

_____	**1.**	Mastoid process	**a.** frontal bone
_____	**2.**	Cribriform plate	**b.** sphenoid bone
_____	**3.**	Infraorbital foramen	**c.** temporal bone
_____	**4.**	The "cheek bone"	**d.** mandible
_____	**5.**	Foramen magnum	**e.** ethmoid bone
_____	**6.**	Coronoid process	**f.** maxillary bone
_____	**7.**	Supraorbital margin	**g.** occipital bone
_____	**8.**	Hypoglossal canal	**h.** zygomatic bone
_____	**9.**	Foramen ovale	
_____	**10.**	Crista galli	
_____	**11.**	Internal acoustic meatus	
_____	**12.**	Hypophyseal fossa	
_____	**13.**	Styloid process	
_____	**14.**	The lower jaw bone	

Labeling

Draw your own lines and then label the following features on the diagram.

a. Xiphoid process   **f.** 5th rib

b. Head of radius   **g.** Coronoid fossa

c. Greater tubercle   **h.** Jugular notch

d. Capitulum   **i.** Acromion process

e. Coracoid process

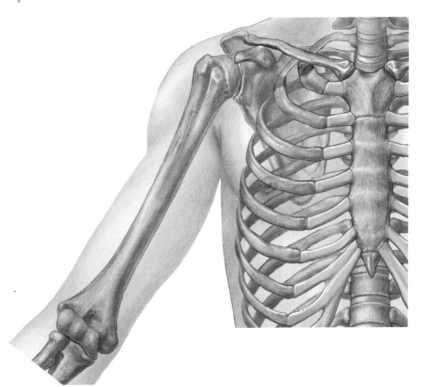

Draw your own lines and then label the following features on the diagram.

a. Medial malleolus
b. Patella
c. Head of fibula
d. 5th metatarsal
e. Talus

f. Tibial tuberosity
g. Intercondylar eminence
h. Cuboid
i. Lateral condyle of femur

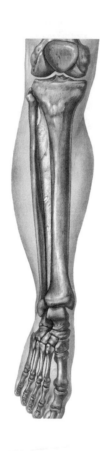

Draw your own lines and then label the following features on the diagram.

a.	Ventral sacral foramina	**g.**	12th rib
b.	Anterior superior iliac spine	**h.**	Pubic symphysis
c.	Obturator foramen	**i.**	Ischial tuberosity
d.	Body of L3 vertebra	**j.**	Coccyx
e.	Greater trochanter	**k.**	Neck of femur
f.	Iliac crest		

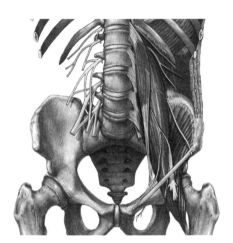

Fill in the Blank/Short Answer

1. The two bones that make up the nasal septum are the _____ and _____.

2. The four skull bones that contain paranasal sinuses are the _____,

    _____, _____, and _____.

3. The fontanelles of the skull typically close by what age? _____

4. The cervical spine contains _____ vertebrae, the thoracic spine contains

    _____ vertebrae, and the lumbar spine has _____.

5. The second cervical vertebra is also known as the _____.

6. A lateral curvature of the spine is known as _____.

7. The clavicle articulates medially with the _____ and laterally with the _____.

8. Ribs 8 to 10 are known as _____ or _____ ribs.

9. The _____ border of the scapula is also known as the axillary border.

10. The _____ of the humerus articulates with the _____ of the radius.

11. Digit 1 of the hand is also known as the thumb or _____.

12. The three bones that fuse to form the hip bone or os coxae are the _____,

    _____, and _____.

13. When an elderly person with osteoporosis "breaks the hip," the bone (and feature) that the person actually breaks is really the _____.

14. The bumps that most people refer to as the ankle are actually called the medial and lateral _____.

15. The great toe is properly known as the _____, while the heel bone is more correctly called the _____.

Essay

1. Describe the normal developmental process of the primary and secondary curvatures of the spine and give some examples of abnormal curvatures.

2. Compare and contrast several characteristics of osteoarthritis and rheumatoid arthritis.

Muscular System

LEARNING OBJECTIVES

Upon completion of this chapter, the student should be able to:

- Describe the major functions of the muscular system
- Describe common muscle origins and insertions as well as synergists and antagonists for major muscle groups
- Provide examples of criteria used when naming muscles
- Locate and identify the major muscles of the head and neck
- Locate and identify the major muscles of the chest and back
- Locate and identify the major muscles of the upper extremity
- Locate and identify the major muscles of the lower extremity

MUSCULAR SYSTEM OVERVIEW

Of the three types of muscle tissue in the body (skeletal, cardiac, and smooth), skeletal muscle is the only type to be under voluntary control. While all three muscle types can contract and produce movement, it is skeletal muscle that is primarily responsible for the movement of the body. Skeletal muscle allows for locomotion (walking) as well as smaller, more coordinated movements such as writing, driving, and even smiling. Some skeletal muscles are arranged in circular patterns around hollow passages (sphincters) controlling the movement of substances along those passages such as with urination and defecation. Skeletal muscles are continuously making small adjustments here and there to help us maintain our posture and hold our body position (so you do not fall out of your seat while reading this). As muscles use ATP for energy, they give off heat as a by-product of muscle contraction. This heat then helps us to maintain our normal body temperature. If you have ever experienced shivering, you know your muscles will contract involuntarily when you get cold in an attempt to help warm your body. Skeletal muscles can also help provide some protection. They have a limited ability to protect internal organs, such as those in the abdominal cavity. Also, while the action of many muscles is to cause movement at joints, they can also serve to stabilize and protect the joints. While a strain is damage to a muscle or tendon, a sprain is damage to a ligament that connects bone to bone. It is common practice to strengthen surrounding muscles after a sprain (of the knee, for example) in an attempt to stabilize the affected joint.

NAMING SKELETAL MUSCLES

At first glance, it may appear that muscles have some pretty outrageous names, but by understanding some key characteristics, naming muscles will seem a bit more practical. Some muscles are named based on their relative **size** such as maximus (biggest), minimus (smallest), longus (longest), and brevis (shortest). Some muscles are named based on their **shape** such as the deltoid (for the Greek letter delta, meaning triangle), rhomboid, and trapezius. Muscles may also be named for the **number of origins** they contain. The biceps brachii on the anterior arm has two origins, while the triceps brachii on the posterior arm has three origins. The quadriceps group of the thigh consists of four muscles that work together to extend the knee. Some muscles are named for the **actions** they perform such as the adductors of the thigh, the levator scapulae (elevation of the scapula), flexor carpi radialis (wrist flexion), or the depressor anguli oris (pulls down the corner of the mouth). Muscles may be named for the **orientation of the fibers** such as the rectus (straight) femoris of the thigh or the external oblique (on a slant) of the abdomen. Finally, some muscles are named for the **location** of the muscle or by their attachment sites (origin and insertion). The sternocleidomastoid muscle has its origin from the sternum (sterno) and clavicle (cleido) and its insertion into the mastoid process of the temporal bone. The epicranius may be found "upon the cranium" and consists of the frontalis over the frontal bone and the occipitalis over the occipital bone.

Every one of our skeletal muscles attaches to either bone or another form of connective tissue. **Tendons** are cord-like structures that serve to attach muscle to bone, whereas **aponeuroses** are flat, sheet-like collections of connective tissue that serve as a more broad area of muscular attachment. The point of attachment that is more stable and often immovable is called the **origin**. The attachment site that is more moveable is referred to as the **insertion**. Since skeletal muscle cannot push and must always pull, or shorten, as the muscle contracts, the insertion then moves toward the origin. The major muscle that is responsible for a particular action is called the **agonist**, or **prime mover**. Muscles that assist the prime mover by reinforcing the same action at that joint are called **synergists**, whereas muscles that cause the opposite action on the same joint are referred to as **antagonists**. The biceps brachii is considered a prime mover for elbow flexion and the brachialis would function as a synergist helping to reinforce the same action, whereas the triceps brachii would be an antagonistic muscle opposing elbow flexion. Antagonists may sometimes serve as prime movers as well. While the triceps brachii is an antagonist for elbow flexion, it is considered the prime mover for elbow extension.

CLINICAL APPLICATIONS

Sprains and strains are common (and painful) musculoskeletal injuries, but what is the difference between the two? A sprain is damage to a ligament that connects bone to bone, whereas a strain is damage that occurs to either a muscle or the tendon that connects the muscle to bone. Because muscle tissue is more vascular than connective tissue, strains tend to heal more rapidly, and completely, than sprains. Because sprains may lead to joint instability, it is also more common for them to reoccur as compared to strains. Proper warm-up exercises and stretching can help minimize the risk of musculoskeletal injury with activity.

To view the image in AIA:
1. *Click on Clinical Illustrations; Select "**All**," "**Muscular**," "**All**," "**All**," and "**All**" from the associated drop-down menus.*
2. *Click "**Search**."*
3. *Find the images titled **Tendon versus ligament** and **Flexibility exercise**.*

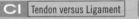 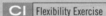

LAB ACTIVITY 2.1

Muscles of the Head and Neck

The muscles of the head and neck have some unique characteristics. For example, many facial muscles insert into the skin, rather than bone. This allows us to portray our wide range of emotion with facial expressions. Other muscles, such as the **masseter** and **temporalis**, serve to help us chew our food and are called muscles of **mastication**. The neck muscles, such as the **sternocleidomastoid**, often have attachments to the trunk or shoulder girdle and allow us to enjoy the wide range of motion we see with our head.

Identify and label the frontalis, orbicularis oculi, orbicularis oris, levator labii superioris, zygomaticus major/ minor, and sternocleidomastoid in the figure below. To view the image in AIA, go to

  or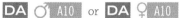

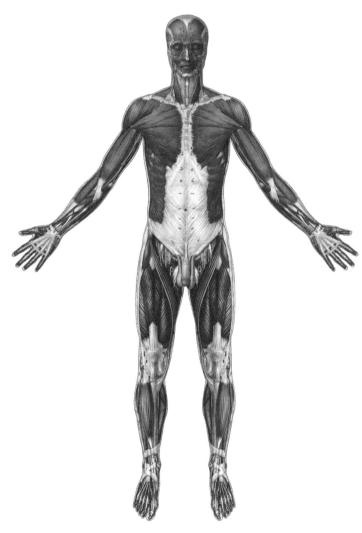

The two major muscles of mastication, the masseter and temporalis, may be seen and labeled in the lateral view below. The temporalis is visible deep to the fascia. You may also view and label the occipitalis connecting to the frontalis via the galea aponeurotica. The depressor anguli oris and depressor labii inferioris may also be visualized and labeled in the following view.

  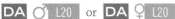 or

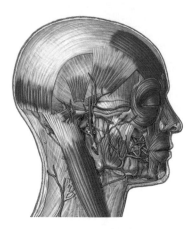

 LAB ACTIVITY 2.2

Muscles of the Trunk and Arm

The muscles of the trunk have a wide array of functions. Many of the muscles help to move the head and neck as well as the upper limb, including those that stabilize the scapulae. Since several muscles of the trunk cross the shoulder joint and act on the humerus, they will be considered in this section as well. The major, superficial muscle of the chest is the **pectoralis major**. The major muscle of the anterior arm, the **biceps brachii**, crosses both the shoulder and the elbow joints and allows for flexion of both joints. Antagonistic to the biceps brachii, the **triceps brachii** is the posterior arm counterpart. The **deltoid** muscle has anterior and posterior attachments to the shoulder girdle and is the main abductor of the arm. The **intercostal** muscles, along with the **pectoralis minor**, act on the ribs to aid with respiration. The superficial, posterior muscles of the back are made up of the more superior **trapezius** and the inferior **latissimus dorsi** muscles. Deep posterior muscles help to support and move the vertebral column. While the abdominal muscles act on the vertebral column as well, they also offer some protection of the underlying viscera of the abdominal cavity.

Identify and label the superficial anterior muscles including the deltoid, pectoralis major, biceps brachii, and sternocleidomastoid in the figure below. The external oblique and the origin of the serratus anterior may also be seen here. To view the image in AIA, go to

  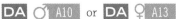 or

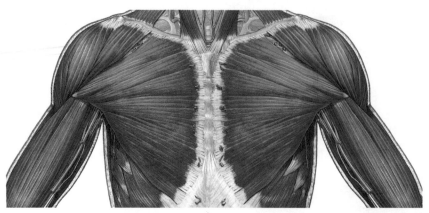

With the pectoralis major removed, you can easily view and label the smaller, deeper pectoralis minor in the following figure. Additionally you can distinguish between the short and long heads of the biceps brachii from this view. To view the image in AIA, go to

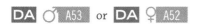

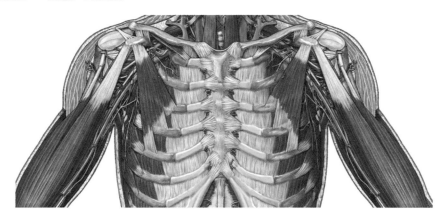

Moving just a bit deeper you can visualize and label the remaining two muscles of the anterior arm. The coracobrachialis is the proximal muscle that crosses the shoulder joint, while the brachialis is the more distal muscle that crosses the elbow joint. To view the image in AIA, go to

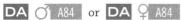

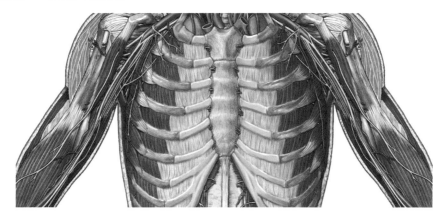

LAB ACTIVITY 2.3

Switching to the posterior view allows you to visualize the superficial muscles of the back. Using the "zoom-out" function in AIA allows you to visualize the entire back, whereas the "zoom-in" will allow you to view the upper and lower back separately.

In the figure below, you can easily visualize and label the large trapezius and latissimus dorsi muscles. You may also see the splenius capitis, deltoid, infraspinatus, and the teres major and minor muscles. The muscle covering the posterior aspect of the arm is the triceps brachii. To view the image in AIA, go to

   or

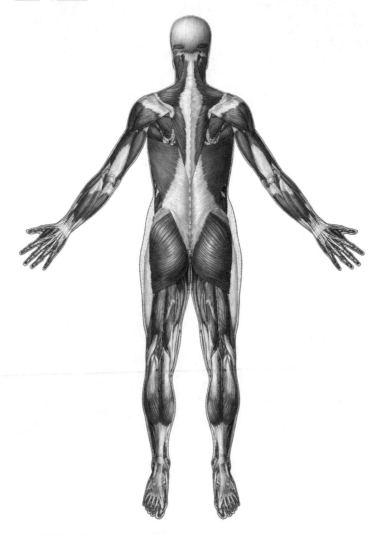

LAB ACTIVITY 2.4

Removing the trapezius and latissimus dorsi allows you to view some of the deeper muscles of the back. The deep group of muscles known as the **erector spinae**, or **sacrospinalis**, runs the entire length of the spinal column from the ilium to the skull. They include the **iliocostalis**, **longissimus**, and **spinalis** muscles. Many muscles that attach to the scapula may also now be seen. The *rotator cuff* is a group of four muscles that originate on the scapula and insert into the humerus. Three of the four muscles may be seen from the posterior view. They are the **supraspinatus**, **infraspinatus**, and **teres minor**. The fourth muscle, the **subscapularis**, must be viewed from the anterior aspect of the scapula. The larger **teres major**, which is not part of the rotator cuff, may be seen inferior to the teres minor as it is separated from the teres minor by the long head of the **triceps brachii**. The **rhomboid major** and **minor** are found lying between the spinal column and the medial border of the scapula. The **levator scapulae** may be seen arising from the upper cervical vertebrae and inserting into the superior angle of the scapula.

To locate the intermediate back muscle image in AIA:
1. *Click on **Atlas Anatomy**; Select "**Body Wall and Back**," "**Muscular**," "**Posterior**," and "**Illustration**" from the associated drop-down menus.*
2. *Click "**Search**."*
3. *Find the image titled **Intermediate Muscles of Back**.*

AA | Intermediate Muscles of Back

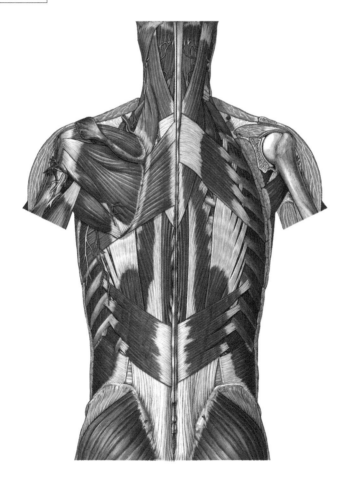

LAB ACTIVITY 2.5

Muscles of the Forearm and Hand

The majority of muscles that move the hand and wrist originate from the humerus and forearm. Wrist and finger flexors tend to originate from the medial epicondyle of the humerus, while wrist and finger extensors originate from the lateral epicondyle. Overuse of these particular muscles often leads to tennis elbow (medial epicondylitis) and golfers elbow (lateral epicondylitis), respectively. The muscles of the anterior forearm can be divided into three layers as evidenced by the following three images.

Find and label the brachioradialis, pronator teres, flexor carpi radialis, palmaris longus, and flexor carpi ulnaris in the following image: To view the image in AIA, go to

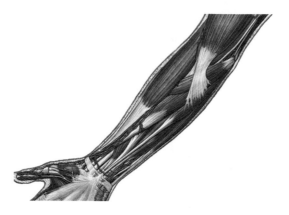 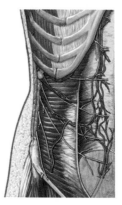

The middle layer of the anterior forearm shows the flexor digitorum superficialis. To view the image in AIA, go to

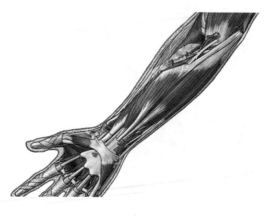 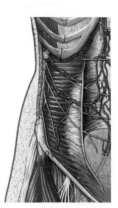

The deep layer of the anterior forearm shows the flexor pollicis longus laterally and the flexor digitorum profundus medially, overlying the pronator quadratus muscle. To view the image in AIA, go to

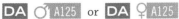 or

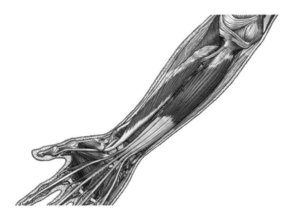 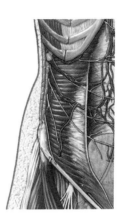

LAB ACTIVITY 2.6

From the posterior view of the forearm, the following extensor muscles may be visualized: **extensor carpi radialis longus**, **extensor carpi radialis brevis**, **extensor digitorum**, and **extensor carpi ulnaris**. The flexor carpi ulnaris may also be seen from this view, but it should be noted that it originates from the medial epicondyle of the humerus, whereas the extensor muscles originate from the lateral epicondyle.

Find and label the wrist and finger extensor musculature in the following image: To view the image in AIA, go to

 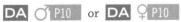 or

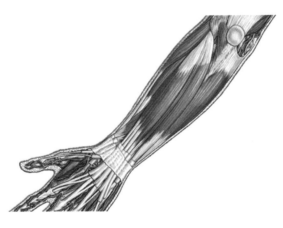 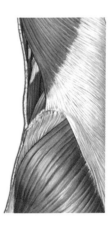

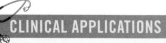

CLINICAL APPLICATIONS

Most people recognize that **strength training** is an important component of most fitness plans, but nonetheless there are many misconceptions with regard to the effects of strength training. You will hear people say "I don't want to lift weights because I don't want to get all big and bulky" or "I only want to do aerobic exercise since I am trying to lose weight and muscle weighs more than fat" or the ever popular "Once you stop lifting weights all of that extra muscle turns into fat." *So what really happens when you strength train or after you stop?* First, rest assured that it is quite difficult to get big and bulky. It takes a lot of hard work and a lot of time. While circuit training and many common resistance-type exercises performed in most commercial fitness centers will serve to make muscles stronger and increase muscle tone, generally those types of exercise routines do NOT make you big and bulky. Secondly, fat and muscle weigh the same: 5 pounds of fat weighs the same as 5 pounds of muscle. The difference is that muscle tissue is more dense than fat and therefore occupies less space—a wonderful attribute for those trying to slim down. It is often recommended that those trying to lose weight should judge their progress more by the fit of their clothes than the number on the scale. If the scale is not changing as much you would like but your clothes are fitting more loosely, you can be assured that your body is changing. Additionally, muscle tissue is more metabolically active than fat; that is, it requires more energy (*calories*) to maintain than does fat. As a result, individuals with more muscle mass burn more calories at rest than individuals with a higher percentage of body fat, helping them to maintain a more healthful weight. Lastly, recall from your study of histology that there are four major classifications of tissues in the body: **epithelial, nervous, muscle**, and **connective**. Fat (adipose tissue) is classified as connective tissue. Tissue types are unable to transform from one classification to another, making it impossible for muscle tissue to "turn into fat" once you stop exercising. Unused muscle can become weaker, **atrophy** (shrink), and exhibit less muscle tone than active muscle, but it cannot change into fat. It is always a good idea to consult a trained professional when embarking on a physical fitness regimen to be assured that your plan is safe and in line with your health goals.

To view some images of muscle and fat tissue, muscle atrophy, and a summary of the four tissue classifications in AIA:
1. *Click on Clinical Illustrations; Select "**All**," "**Muscular**," "**All**," "**All**," and "**Physiology**" from the associated drop-down menus.*
2. *Click "**Search**."*
3. *Find the corresponding images.*

 LAB ACTIVITY 2.7

Muscles of the Hip and Thigh

The muscles that act on the hip joint originate on the pelvis and insert into the femur. Anteriorly, the **iliacus** and **psoas major** serve as hip flexors and share a common insertion known as the *iliopsoas*. Of the four muscles that make the group known as the *quadriceps*, only the rectus femoris crosses the hip joint. Together with the **rectus femoris**, the **vastus lateralis**, **vastus intermedius**, and **vastus medialis** all act to extend the leg at the knee. The **sartorius** is the long, strap-like muscle found overlying the quadriceps. It crosses, and acts upon, both the hip and knee joints. The only major muscle on the lateral thigh is the **tensor fasciae latae,** which may be seen inserting into the long, white band of connective tissue known as the **iliotibial tract** or **iliotibial band (ITB)**. The medial thigh houses the group of muscles known as *adductors,* which includes the **gracilis** or groin muscle. The posterior hip (buttocks) is the location of the **gluteal** muscles (**maximus, medius**, and **minimus**) as well as the deeper **piriformis** and **quadratus femoris**. The group of muscles found on the posterior thigh is known as the *hamstrings*. All three muscles originate from the ischial tuberosity and then cross, and act on, both the hip and knee joints. The hamstring group includes the **biceps femoris, semitendinosus**, and **semimembranosus**.

Find and label the deep hip flexor musculature in the following image: To view the image in AIA, go to

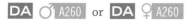 or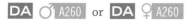

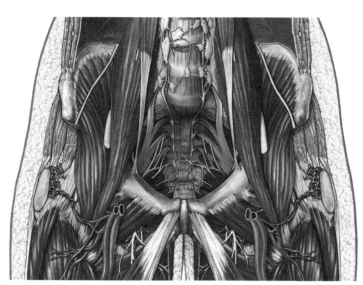

Find and label the muscles of the anterior thigh, as well as the tensor fasciae latae, in the following image: To view the image in AIA, go to

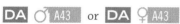

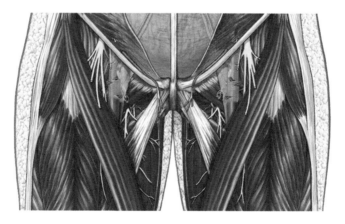

Going a bit deeper, removing the rectus femoris, allows for visualization of the vastus intermedius. To view the image in AIA, go to

 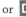 or

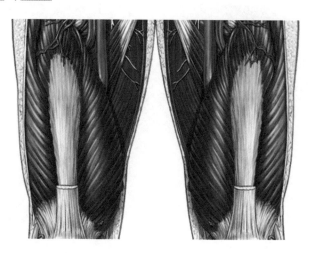

 LAB ACTIVITY 2.8

To locate and label the muscles of the posterior hip and thigh in AIA:
1. *Click on* **Atlas Anatomy**; *Select* "**Lower Limb**," "**Muscular**," "**Posterior**," *and* "**Illustration**" *from the associated drop-down menus.*
2. *Click* "**Search**."
3. *Find the image titled* **Posterior Thigh.**

AA Posterior Thigh

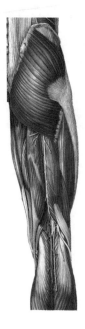

To view and label the deep gluteal muscles image in AIA:
1. Click on **Atlas Anatomy**; Select "**Lower limb**," "**Muscular**," "**Posterior**," and "**Illustration**" from the associated drop-down menus.
2. Click "**Search**."
3. Find the image titled **Gluteal Region (Post)**.

AA | Gluteal Region (Post)

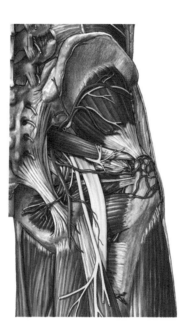

The adductor muscles of the thigh may be viewed and labeled in the following image in AIA:
1. Click on **Atlas Anatomy**; Select "**Lower limb**," "**Muscular**," "**Medial**," and "**Illustration**" from the associated drop-down menus.
2. Click "**Search**."
3. Find the image titled **Medial Thigh**.

AA | Medial Thigh

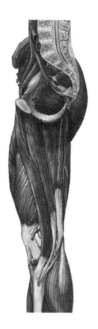

LAB ACTIVITY 2.9

Muscles of the Leg and Foot

The majority of muscles that act on the ankle and toes actually originate on the leg. The anterior leg muscles act to invert and dorsiflex the ankle and extend the toes. They are the **tibialis anterior**, the **extensor hallucis longus**, and the **extensor digitorum longus**. The muscles of the lateral leg serve to evert the ankle and include the **peroneus (fibularis) longus** and the **peroneus (fibularis) brevis**. The posterior leg muscles are divided into a superficial and a deep group and serve to plantarflex the ankle and flex the toes. The superficial group is referred to as the *triceps surae* and includes the **gastrocnemius** (medial and lateral heads) and the **soleus**. These muscles share a common tendon of insertion into the calcaneus, namely, the **calcaneal (Achilles) tendon**. The deep muscles of the posterior leg from medial to lateral include the **flexor digitorum longus**, **posterior tibialis**, and **flexor hallucis longus**.

Find and label the musculature of the anterior leg in the following image: To view the image in AIA, go to

  A43 or   A43

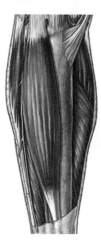 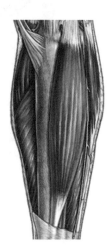

Find and label the muscles of the lateral leg in the following image: To view the image in AIA, go to

  L60 or   L60

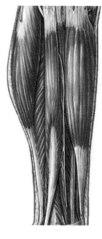

Find and label the musculature of the superficial posterior leg in the following image: To view the image in AIA, go to

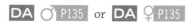 or

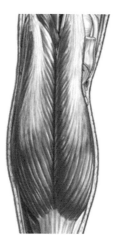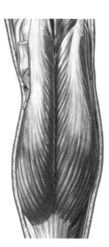

Going a bit deeper, removing the triceps surae, allows for visualization of the deep posterior leg muscles. To view the image in AIA, go to

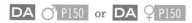 or

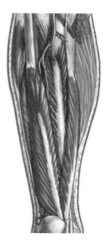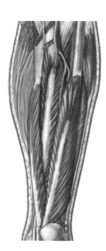

MUSCULAR SYSTEM REVIEW EXERCISES

Matching

_____ **1.** Muscle named for orientation of fibers

_____ **2.** Muscle named for location

_____ **3.** Muscle named for number of origins

_____ **4.** Muscle named for shape

_____ **5.** Muscle named for its origin and insertion

_____ **6.** Muscle named for its size

_____ **7.** Muscle named for its action

    a. depressor anguli oris

    b. trapezius

    c. rectus femoris

    d. tibialis anterior

    e. triceps brachii

    f. coracobrachialis

    g. gluteus minimus

Labeling

Draw your own lines and then label following features on the diagram.

    a. Pectoralis major

    b. Frontalis

    c. Sternocleidomastoid

    d. Orbicularis oculi

    e. Brachioradialis

    f. Deltoid

    g. Biceps brachii

    h. Serratus anterior

    i. Pronator teres

    j. Orbicularis oris

    k. External oblique

    l. Palmaris longus

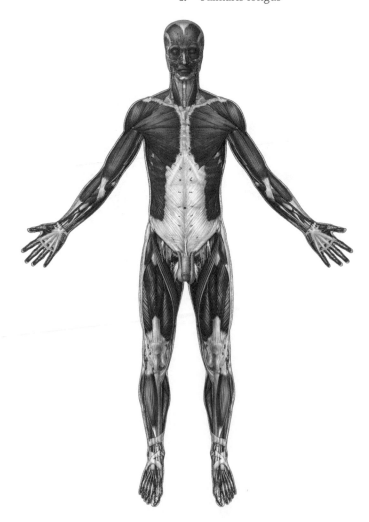

Draw your own lines and then label following features on the diagram.

a. Latissimus dorsi
b. Splenius capitis
c. Gluteus maximus
d. Trapezius

e. Triceps brachii
f. Teres major
g. Extensor digitorum
h. Deltoid

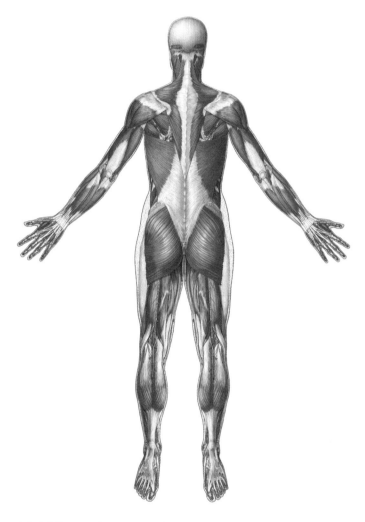

Draw your own lines and then label following features on the diagram.

a. Vastus lateralis
b. Tibialis anterior
c. Sartorius
d. Tensor fascia latae

e. Adductor longus
f. Rectus femoris
g. Iliotibial tract
h. Vastus medialis

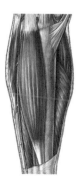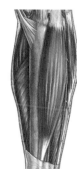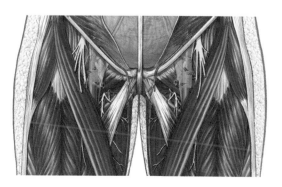

Fill in the Blank/Short Answer

1. A muscle that opposes a muscle action at a joint is called a(n) _____.

2. The muscular attachment that is the more moveable end is known as the _____.

3. A circular muscle that helps regulate the movement of materials through passageways is known as a

   _____.

4. Lateral epicondylitis is also known as _____.

5. A broad, flat connective tissue attachment for muscles is known as a(n) _____.

6. The connective tissue attachment that connects bones to bones is known as a

   _____.

7. Another name for the calcaneal tendon is the _____ tendon.

8. The iliopsoas is the combination of which two muscles? _____.

9. The four muscles of the rotator cuff are: _____ _____.

10. The only muscle of the quadriceps group to cross the hip joint is the _____.

11. Name a muscle that is used to make a fist. _____.

12. Name a muscle that is used to stand on your tiptoes. _____.

Essay

1. Describe at least five functions of the muscular system.

2. Give a prime mover, synergist, and antagonist for elbow flexion.

3. Give a prime mover, synergist, and antagonist for plantarflexion of the ankle.

Nervous System

LEARNING OBJECTIVES

Upon completion of this chapter, the student should be able to:

- Locate and identify the major surface features and internal features of the brain

- Provide examples of functions for the common brain regions

- Understand the flow of cerebrospinal fluid through the brain and spinal cord

- Describe and label the cross-sectional anatomy of the spinal cord as well as the meninges that surround the central nervous system

- Locate and identify the four spinal nerve plexuses and identify the major nerves arising from each

- Understand the origin of the two divisions of the autonomic nervous system and identify some structures that are unique to each division

- Be familiar with a few common pathologies of the nervous system

NERVOUS SYSTEM OVERVIEW

The nervous system is often referred to as the "master system" of the body because it controls and coordinates the actions of all of our body systems. The nervous system receives information from all parts of the body via nerve impulses, interprets that information, and then provides for a response to be made through its communication with the various muscles, glands, and organs of the body. The two major divisions of the nervous system include the central nervous system and the peripheral nervous system.

The **central nervous system (CNS)** consists of the **brain** and **spinal cord** and is responsible for integration and interpretation of incoming sensory information as well as initiating a response to that information.

The **peripheral nervous system (PNS)** consists of nerves and specialized nerve receptors that lie outside of the CNS. The PNS is made up of 12 pairs of **cranial nerves** that connect to the brain and 31 pairs of **spinal nerves** that connect to the spinal cord. These nerves serve as two-way communication lines between all of the tissues of the body and the CNS.

The PNS has two subdivisions based on the functions carried out by the nerves. The **sensory (afferent) division** consists of nerves that convey electrical impulses to the CNS from peripheral receptors located throughout the body. Sensory fibers from the skin, muscles, and joints are referred to as *somatic sensory*, while fibers from visceral organs and glands are referred to as *visceral sensory*.

The **motor (efferent) division** carries nerve impulses from the CNS to the muscles, organs, and glands of the body and is itself further subdivided into two divisions. The **somatic (voluntary) system** is so named because it controls the skeletal muscles of the body which are under voluntary control. The **autonomic (involuntary) system (ANS)** controls smooth and cardiac muscle, glands, and organs that are under involuntary control. Finally, the autonomic nervous system has two divisions—the **sympathetic division** and the **parasympathetic division**. While both divisions serve many of the same organs, they often have opposing effects.

LAB ACTIVITY 3.1

External Brain Features

The human brain is divided into several major regions: the **cerebrum**, **diencephalon**, **brainstem**, and **cerebellum**. The cerebrum is the largest, most superior region of the brain and consists of paired **cerebral hemispheres** containing many bumps and grooves. The raised projections are referred to as *gyri* while the shallow grooves are referred to as *sulci*. A few deeper grooves, called *fissures*, may also be seen. The **longitudinal fissure** lies in the midsagittal plane and separates the left and right hemispheres. The cerebrum may be divided into four lobes named for the skull bones that lie over them: the frontal, parietal, temporal, and occipital. The **central sulcus** separates the **frontal lobe** from the **parietal lobe**. Anterior to the central sulcus is the **precentral gyrus,** which is the *primary motor area* of the brain, while the **postcentral gyrus** lies posterior to the central sulcus and is known as the *primary somatic sensory area*. The **lateral sulcus** separates the **temporal lobe** from the **parietal lobe**. The temporal lobe contains the auditory area of the brain, whereas the most posterior lobe of the cerebrum, the **occipital lobe**, contains the *visual area*. From the external view of the brain, the **cerebellum** is also visible. The cerebellum also has two hemispheres and is responsible for maintaining balance and coordination of skeletal muscles. The inferior most aspect of the brainstem, the **pons** and **medulla oblongata**, are also visible from the exterior. The brainstem contains many autonomic nuclei that control functions such as those associated with the respiratory and cardiovascular systems. *For a unique interactive experience, click on the 3D Anatomy icon and then select 3D Brain. From there you are able to manipulate a three-dimensional brain by rotating it, moving it, and zooming in and out of it.*

Identify and label the external features of the brain in the following figure.
To locate the image in AIA:
1. *Click on **Atlas Anatomy**; Select "**Head and Neck**," "**Nervous**," "**Lateral**," and "**Illustration**" from the associated drop-down menus.*
2. *Click "**Search**."*
3. *Find the image titled **Brain (Lat).***

To view a similar image, you may go to **DA** ♂ L191 *or* **DA** ♀ L192

AA | Brain (Lat)

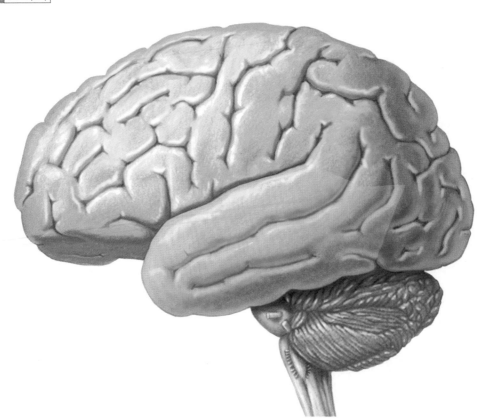

1. *Click on **Clinical Illustrations**; Select "**Head and Neck**," "**Nervous**," "**Lateral**," "**Illustration**," and "**Neurology**" from the associated drop-down menus.*
2. *Click "**Search**."*
3. *Find the image titled **Brain**.*

CI Brain

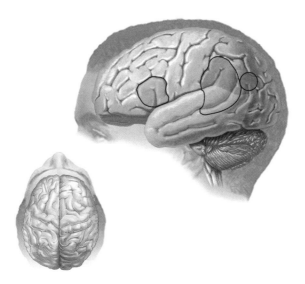

CLINICAL APPLICATIONS

Meningitis is a condition where the protective connective tissue membranes around the brain and spinal cord (meninges) become infected and inflamed. While meningitis may have such causes as physical trauma, cancer, and even certain medications, the most common causes are the result of either bacterial or viral infections. Generally speaking, *viral meningitis* is rarely fatal in a healthy individual. *Bacterial meningitis*, on the other hand, is usually much more serious and requires prompt attention and treatment. In severe cases meningitis may progress to *encephalitis* (inflammation of the brain) and lead to permanent brain damage or even death.

To view an image of the meninges surrounding the brain in AIA:
1. *Click on Clinical Illustrations; Select "**All**," "**Nervous**," "**All**," "**All**," and "**Neurology**" from the associated drop-down menus.*
2. *Click "**Search**."*
3. *Find the corresponding images.*

LAB ACTIVITY 3.2

Internal Brain Features

A midsagittal section of the brain reveals many features not visible from the external view. The large, comma-shaped **corpus callosum** is a collection of fiber tracts that connect the two cerebral hemispheres. Inferior to the corpus callosum is the *diencephalon*. The diencephalon contains three subdivisions that all contain "thalamus" in their name. The **thalamus** is a major relay center where incoming sensory information is directed to the appropriate area of the cerebral cortex for interpretation. The **hypothalamus** is a neuroendocrine structure that is a major visceral control center responsible for regulating body temperature, water balance, satiety, and many other autonomic functions. The hypothalamus also produces several hormones that are stored in the **pituitary gland** or influence the release of its hormones. The hypothalamus connects inferiorly to the pituitary gland via the **infundibulum**. The **epithalamus** contains the *pineal body* which secretes melatonin and has a role in maintaining circadian rhythms. The three divisions of the *brainstem* are the **midbrain**, **pons**, and **medulla oblongata**. The midbrain contains the **cerebral peduncles** which convey ascending and descending tracts between the cerebrum and the spinal cord. The **corpora quadrigemina** contain paired **superior colliculi** (visual reflex area) and **inferior colliculi** (auditory reflex area). The pons contains fiber tracts as well but also has nuclei for the control of respiration. The medulla oblongata is the most inferior aspect of the brainstem and contains many important autonomic nuclei such as those for controlling heart rate, blood pressure, breathing, vomiting, and even swallowing. From this view, the internal structure of the **cerebellum** is evident. The outer cerebellar cortex is made of gray matter while the deeper white matter is referred to as the **arbor vitae** ("tree of life") for its branched, tree-like appearance.

To observe an animated overview of the regions of the brain:
1. Click on **Clinical Animations**; *Select "**All**," "**Nervous**," and "**All**" from the associated drop-down menus.*
*2. Click "**Search**."*
3. Find the animation titled **Brain Components**.

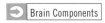 Brain Components

Identify and label the internal features of the brain in the following figure.
To locate the image in AIA:
1. Click on **Atlas Anatomy**; *Select "**Head and Neck**," "**Nervous**," "**Medial**," and "**Illustration**" from the associated drop-down menus.*
*2. Click "**Search**."*
3. Find the image titled **Sagittal Section of Brain**.

To view a similar image, you may go to **DA** ♂ MO *or* **DA** ♀ MO *or click on* **CI** Brain Structures to view an image of labeled internal brain regions.

AA Sagittal Section of Brain

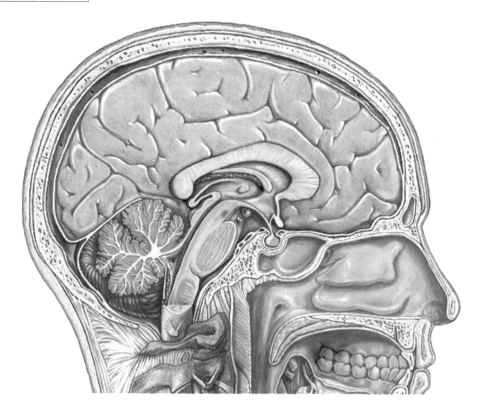

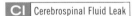

LAB ACTIVITY 3.3

Cerebrospinal Fluid

Cerebrospinal fluid (CSF) is produced by the choroid plexus, specialized capillaries found in each of the four ventricles of the brain. CSF serves to support and cushion the brain and offers protection against trauma to the head. CSF flows from the two lateral ventricles found within the cerebral hemispheres (separated by the septum pellucidum) to the third ventricle (surrounding the diencephalon) via the intraventricular foramen on to the fourth ventricle through the cerebral aqueduct. From the fourth ventricle, CSF flow continues onward through the central canal of the spinal cord and the subarachnoid space surrounding the brain and spinal cord until it is finally reabsorbed into the dural sinuses.

Identify and label the passages associated with the flow of cerebrospinal fluid in the following figure.
To locate the image in AIA:
1. *Click on **Clinical Illustrations**; Select "**Head and Neck**," "**Nervous**," "**Medial**," "**Illustration**," and "**Neurology**" from the associated drop-down menus.*
2. *Click "**Search**."*
3. *Find the image titled **Cerebrospinal Fluid Leak.***

To view the structures in a similar image, you may go to DA ♂ MO *or* DA ♀ MO .

CI | Cerebrospinal Fluid Leak

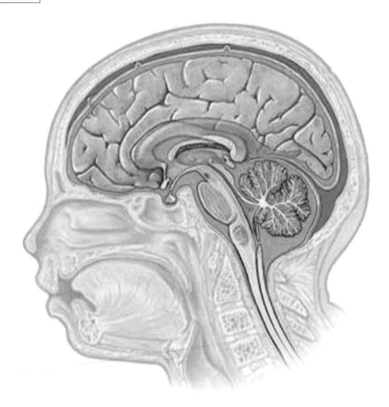

LAB ACTIVITY 3.4

Cranial Nerves

While all 31 pairs of spinal nerves are mixed, that is, they contain both sensory and motor fibers, the 12 pairs of cranial nerves are divided into mixed, sensory, and motor nerves. Cranial nerves are identified by both name and number (Roman numeral) and are visible from the inferior aspect of the brain. The 12 cranial nerves are as follows:

CN I—Olfactory: Sensory nerve for olfaction (smell)

CN II—Optic: Sensory nerve for vision

CN III—Oculomotor: Motor nerve for extraocular eye muscles; parasympathetic fibers to the iris of the eye

CN IV—Trochlear: Motor to the superior oblique muscle of the eye

CN V—Trigeminal: Mixed nerve supplying motor function to the muscles of mastication and sensory fibers from the skin of the face. Three divisions: ophthalmic, maxillary, mandibular

CN VI—Abducens: Motor to the lateral rectus muscle of the eye

CN VII—Facial: Mixed nerve supplying motor fibers to the muscles of facial expression and sensory fibers from the anterior 2/3 of the tongue; parasympathetic fibers to the lacrimal and salivary glands (submandibular and sublingual)

CN VIII—Vestibulocochlear: Sensory nerve for hearing and equilibrium

CN IX—Glossopharyngeal: Mixed nerve supplying motor fibers to the pharyngeal muscles and sensory fibers from the posterior 1/3 of the tongue; parasympathetic fibers to parotid salivary gland

CN X—Vagus: Motor and sensory fibers to the pharynx and larynx; parasympathetic fibers to/from heart, lungs, esophagus, stomach, small intestine, proximal large intestine, liver, pancreas, gallbladder

CN XI—(Spinal) Accessory: Motor fibers to the sternocleidomastoid and trapezius muscles

CN XII—Hypoglossal: Motor fibers to muscles of the tongue

Identify and label the cranial nerves in the following figure.

To locate the image in AIA:

1. Click on **Atlas Anatomy***; Select* "**Head and Neck**," "**Nervous**," "**Inferior**," *and* "**Illustration**" *from the associated drop-down menus.*

2. Click "**Search**."

3. Find the image titled **Base of Brain (Inf)**

AA Base of Brain (Inf)

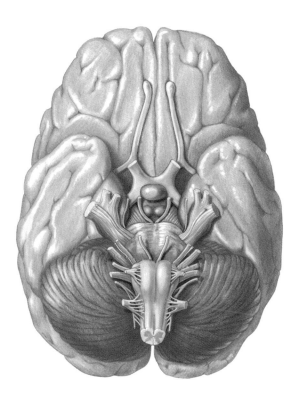

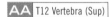
LAB ACTIVITY 3.5

Spinal Cord

The spinal cord is continuous superiorly with the medulla oblongata and descends inferiorly to the level of the L1/L2 intervertebral disc, terminating at the **conus medullaris**. While the spinal cord ends at L1/L2, spinal nerves continue to occupy the remainder of the vertebral canal. The appearance of those nerves resembles a horse's tail and is aptly named the **cauda equina**. The conus medullaris is anchored to the sacrum by a pia mater extension known as the **filum terminale**. The cross-sectional anatomy of the cord is composed of both white and gray matter. The outer white matter consists of ascending and descending nerve tracts divided into areas referred to as **anterior, lateral, and posterior funiculi**. The inner gray matter resembles the letter "H" and is divided into "horns." The **dorsal horn** contains cell bodies of sensory neurons while the **ventral horn** contains those of somatomotor fibers. Spinal cord levels T1 through L2 and S2 to S4 also contain a lateral horn. The **lateral horns** of T1 to L2 contain cell bodies of autonomic motor fibers of the sympathetic nervous system while those of S2 to S4 contain cell bodies of parasympathetic fibers.

The spinal cord gives rise to 31 pairs of mixed spinal nerves. Both somatic motor and autonomic motor fibers exit the spinal cord via the **ventral root**. Cell bodies of somatic sensory fibers are found within the **dorsal root ganglion** and together with autonomic sensory fibers enter the spinal cord via the **dorsal root**. The **spinal nerve** is found where the ventral and dorsal roots unite. As the spinal nerve exits the intervertebral foramen, it separates into two divisions. The smaller, **dorsal ramus** stays relatively local and supplies the skin and deep muscles of the back, whereas the larger **ventral ramus** continues to either merge with adjacent segments to form a nerve **plexus** or continue on as an **intercostal nerve** to serve the muscles of the thorax.

Identify and label the cross-sectional features of the spinal cord in the following figure.
To locate the image in AIA:
1. *Click on **Atlas Anatomy**; Select **"Body Wall and Back," "Nervous," "Superior,"** and **"Illustration"** from the associated drop-down menus.*
2. *Click **"Search."***
3. *Find the image titled **T12 Vertebra (Sup)**.*

AA T12 Vertebra (Sup)

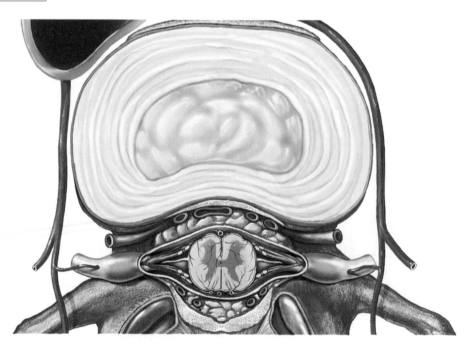

LAB ACTIVITY 3.6

The spinal cord is surrounded and protected by the same three meningeal layers that envelope the brain. The **pia mater** is the deepest layer that is in intimate contact with the central nervous tissue. The middle layer is known as the **arachnoid mater**, whereas the outer fibrous layer is the dura mater. The **dura mater** is a double-layered membrane that anchors to the skull and vertebral canal. The dural layers separate in the brain to contain the **dural sinuses** that collect venous (deoxygenated) blood from the brain.

Identify and label the meninges in the following figure.
To locate the image in AIA:
1. *Click on **Atlas Anatomy**; Select "**Body Wall and Back**," "**Nervous**," "**Non-standard**," and "**Illustration**" from the associated drop-down menus.*
2. *Click "**Search**."*
3. *Find the image titled **Spinal Cord Vessels & Meninges**.*

AA Spinal Cord Vessels & Meninges

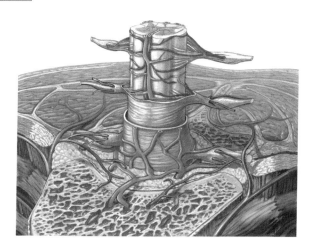

Identify and label the conus medullaris, cauda equina, and filum terminale in the figures below.
To locate the images in AIA:
1. *Click on **Atlas Anatomy**; Select "**Body Wall and Back**," "**Nervous**," "**Posterior**," and "**Illustration**" from the associated drop-down menus.*
2. *Click "**Search**."*
3. *Find the image titled **Lumbosacral Spinal Cord**.*

AA Lumbosacral Spinal Cord

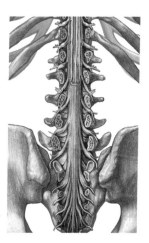

1. Click on **Atlas Anatomy**; Select "**Body Wall and Back**," "**Nervous**," "**Medial**," and "**Illustration**" from the associated drop-down menus.
2. Click "**Search**."
3. Find the image titled **Sagittal Section of Lower Spine**.

AA Sagittal Section of Lower Spine

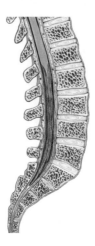

CLINICAL APPLICATIONS

Epidural anesthesia is perhaps the most common form of pain control for women in labor. Epidurals block the sensation of pain from the lower spinal levels and are administered through a catheter fed into the epidural space. The epidural space is the area outside of the dura mater but inside the spinal foramen. The patient is typically in a seated or side-lying "C-shape" position to allow for the opening of the spinal laminae and easier placement of the needle between the vertebrae.

To view the image in AIA:
1. *Click on Clinical Illustrations; Select "**Body Wall and Back**," "**Nervous**," "**Medial**," "**Illustration**," and "**Anesthesiology**" from the associated drop-down menus.*
2. *Click "**Search**."*
3. *Find the images titled **Epidural Needle and Catheter** and **Areas of Numbness in Epidural Anesthesia**.*

CI Epidural Needle and Catheter   **CI** Areas of Numbness in Epidural Anesthesia

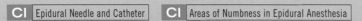

SPINAL NERVES AND NERVE PLEXUSES

As the spinal nerve emerges from the intervertebral foramen, it almost immediately divides into a dorsal and ventral ramus. Since all 31 pairs of spinal nerves are a combination of the ventral and dorsal roots, all rami that branch from those nerves contain both motor and sensory fibers as well. The ventral rami of the cervical, lumbar, and sacral spine form networks known as plexuses which then diverge to form peripheral nerves that serve the upper and lower limbs. In the thoracic spine, the ventral rami continue on without dividing to become intercostal nerves.

LAB ACTIVITY 3.7

Cervical Plexus

The **cervical plexus** arises from the ventral rami of **C1 through C4 (C5)** and supplies the muscles of the neck and shoulder. Perhaps the most important nerve of the cervical plexus is the **phrenic** nerve (C3 to C5), which supplies the diaphragm. Spinal cord trauma superior to C3 may lead to respiratory failure since motor function to the diaphragm may be interrupted.

Identify and label the cervical plexus and phrenic nerve in the following figure.
To locate the image in AIA:
1. Click on ***Atlas Anatomy****; Select* ***"Head and Neck," "Nervous," "Lateral,"*** *and* ***"Illustration"*** *from the associated drop-down menus.*
*2. Click "****Search****."*
3. Find the image titled ***Cervical Plexus (Lat)****.*

AA Cervical Plexus (Lat)

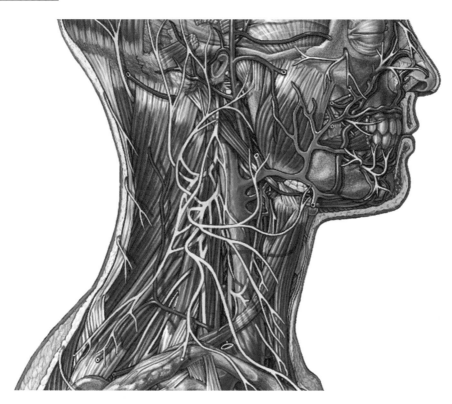

🌿 **LAB ACTIVITY 3.8**

Brachial Plexus

The **brachial plexus** arises from the ventral rami of **C5 to T1** and supplies the muscles of the upper limb via five major nerves. The **axillary** nerve supplies the muscles of the shoulder; the **radial** nerve supplies most of the extensor musculature of the arm and forearm; the **musculocutaneous** nerve supplies the muscles of the arm; the **median** nerve supplies the majority of the wrist flexors on the lateral aspect of the, while the **ulnar** nerve supplies the medial wrist flexors.

Identify and label the brachial plexus and its major nerves in the following figure.
To locate the image in AIA:
1. *Click on **Atlas Anatomy**; Select "**Upper Limb**," "**Nervous**," "**Anterior**," and "**Illustration**" from the associated drop-down menus.*
2. *Click "**Search**."*
3. *Find the image titled **Nerves of Upper Limb (Ant)**.*

AA Nerves of Upper Limb (Ant)

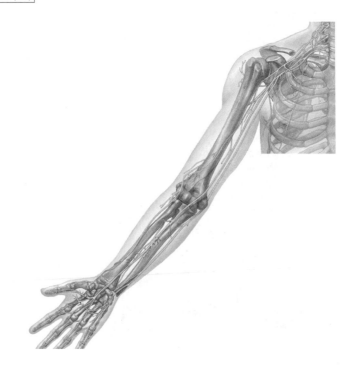

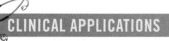

CLINICAL APPLICATIONS

Carpal tunnel syndrome (CTS) is a condition that involves entrapment/impingement of the **median nerve** as it crosses the wrist deep to the *flexor retinaculum*. CTS can result from overuse of the wrist flexors, collapse of the "carpal tunnel," or even as a result of cervical trauma (i.e., whiplash) that causes inflammation of the spinal levels that give rise to the median nerve. CTS usually has both a sensory and motor deficit leading to pain in the wrist and hand in addition to a weakness of wrist and finger flexors. The image below depicts a close-up of the anterior wrist where you may see the structures that occupy the carpal tunnel.

To view the image in AIA:
1. *Click on Atlas Anatomy; Select "**Upper Limb**," "**Nervous**," "**Anterior**," and "**Illustration**," from the associated drop-down menus.*
2. *Click "**Search**."*
3. *Find the image titled **Superficial Palmar Arch 1**.*

AA | Superficial Palmar Arch 1

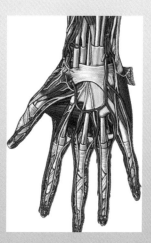

To view the additional CTS specific images in AIA:
1. *Click on Clinical Illustrations; Select "**Upper Limb**," "**Nervous**," "**Anterior**," and "**Illustration**," and "**Neurology**" from the associated drop-down menus.*
2. *Click "**Search**."*
3. *Find the image associated with carpal tunnel syndrome.*

LAB ACTIVITY 3.9

Intercostal Nerves

The ventral rami of the thoracic spine do not contribute to a plexus but rather continue on to become intercostal nerves. The **intercostal nerves** supply the intercostal muscles, which serve to aid in respiration.

Identify and label the intercostal nerves in the following figure.
To locate the image in AIA:
*1. Click on **Atlas Anatomy**; Select "**Body Wall and Back**," "**Nervous**," "**Anterior**," and "**Illustration**" from the associated drop-down menus.*
*2. Click "**Search**."*
*3. Find the image titled **Spinal Nerves of Trunk (Ant)**.*

AA Spinal Nerves of Trunk (Ant)

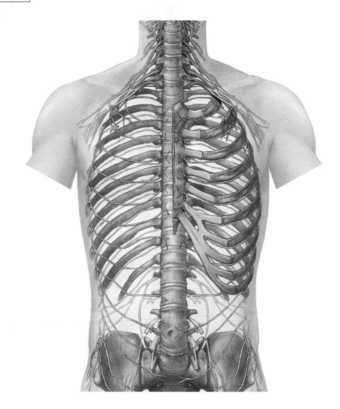

LAB ACTIVITY 3.10

Lumbar Plexus

The **lumbar plexus** arises from the ventral rami of **L1 to L4** and supplies the muscles of the anterior and medial thigh. The **femoral nerve** supplies the anterior thigh muscles while the **obturator nerve** supplies the medial thigh musculature.

Identify and label the lumbar plexus and its major nerves in the following figure.
To locate the image in AIA:
1. *Click on* **Atlas Anatomy**; *Select* "**Lower Limb**," "**Nervous**," "**Anterior**," *and* "**Illustration**" *from the associated drop-down menus.*
2. *Click* "**Search**."
3. *Find the image titled* **Lumbar Plexus In Situ (Ant)**.

AA Lumbar Plexus In Situ (Ant)

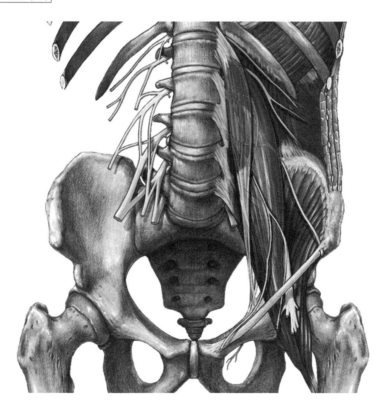

LAB ACTIVITY 3.11

Sacral Plexus

The **sacral plexus** arises from the ventral rami of **L4 to S4** and supplies the muscles of the buttock, posterior thigh, the leg, and foot. The major nerve of the sacral plexus is the sciatic nerve. In the popliteal region, the **sciatic nerve** divides into the **tibial** and **common peroneal** (fibular) nerves that serve to supply the leg and foot.

Identify and label the sacral plexus, the sciatic nerve, and its major branches in the following figure.
To locate the image in AIA:
1. *Click on **Atlas Anatomy**; Select "**Lower Limb**," "**Nervous**," "**Anterior**," and "**Illustration**" from the associated drop-down menus.*
2. *Click "**Search**."*
3. *Find the image titled **Sacral Plexus (Ant)**.*

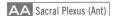 Sacral Plexus (Ant)

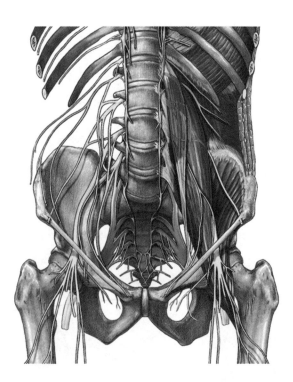

CLINICAL APPLICATIONS

Spina bifida is a congenital condition where the spinous processes of select vertebrae (usually in the lumbar spine) fail to develop. As a result, the laminae are separated by a space where the spinous process should have been. *Spina bifida occulta* (hidden) is a simple nonunion of the laminae that typically has no motor or sensory impairment associated with the condition. Since in many cases it presents with no apparent symptoms, it is often found incidentally when performing tests for other conditions. As such, spina bifida occulta may be diagnosed at most any age. *Meningocele* is a condition associated with spina bifida where parts of the meninges protrude through the gap in the laminae. In these cases, there is a visible sac, usually at the base of the spine, visible at birth. While there is CSF contained in this herniation, there is rarely associated nerve involvement. Prompt surgical correction usually prevents lasting ill effects. *Meningomyelocele* is the most serious condition associated with spina bifida. With meningomyelocele, there is a herniation of spinal nerves in addition to the meninges. In cases of meningomyelocele, there is often related nerve damage and more severe disabilities.

To view an image of spina bifida in AIA:
1. *Click on Clinical Illustrations; Select "All," "Nervous," "All," "All," and "Pediatrics" from the associated drop-down menus.*
2. *Click "Search."*
3. *Find the corresponding image.*

LAB ACTIVITY 3.12

Autonomic Nervous System

The autonomic nervous system (ANS) is the motor division of the peripheral nervous system that controls the automatic (involuntary) functions of the body. The ANS has two major subdivisions—the **sympathetic nervous system (SNS),** which mobilizes the body during extreme situations (stress, excitement, embarrassment), and the **parasympathetic nervous system (PSNS)**, which allows us to conserve energy and control more housekeeping-type activities such as digestion, urination, and defecation. The SNS is also known as the ***thoracolumbar system*** because it arises from the lateral horns of spinal cord levels T1 to L2. The PSNS is known as the ***craniosacral division*** because it arises from cranial nerves III, VII, IX, and X, as well as spinal cord levels S2 to S4. While in most cases organs are innervated by both systems, it is common for one system to be more dominant than the other. In the case of "dual innervation," it is customary for each of the ANS divisions to exert opposing and opposite effects.

Identify the origin and distribution of the sympathetic and parasympathetic nervous systems in the following images.

To locate the images in AIA:

1. *Click on **Atlas Anatomy**; Select "**Abdomen**," "**Nervous**," "**Non-standard**," and "**Illustration**" from the associated drop-down menus.*
2. *Click "**Search**."*
3. *Find the images titled **Autonomic NS-Viscera 1**.*

AA Autonomic NS-Viscera 1   AA Autonomic NS-Viscera 2

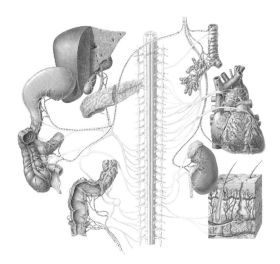
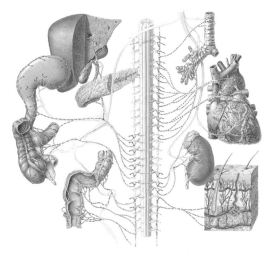

NERVOUS SYSTEM REVIEW EXERCISES

Matching

_____ **1.** Occipital lobe

_____ **2.** Lateral sulcus

_____ **3.** Temporal lobe

_____ **4.** Postcentral gyrus

_____ **5.** Central sulcus

_____ **6.** Precentral gyrus

a. separates the frontal and parietal lobes

b. the primary auditory cortex area

c. the primary visual cortex

d. separates the temporal and parietal lobes

e. the primary somatomotor

f. the primary somatic sensory area

Labeling

Draw your own lines and then label following features on the diagram.

a. Epithalamus

b. Inferior colliculus

c. Pituitary gland

d. Corpus callosum

e. Thalamus

f. Superior colliculus

g. Medulla oblongata

h. Hypothalamus

i. Arbor vitae

j. Pons

k. Infundibulum

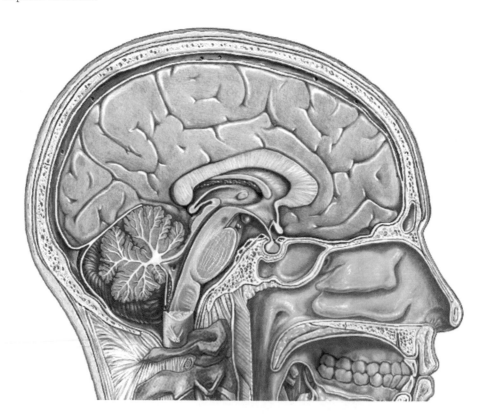

Draw your own lines and then label following features on the diagram.

   a. Third ventricle   **d.** Superior sagittal sinus

   b. Septum pellucidum   **e.** Fourth ventricle

   c. Cerebral aqueduct

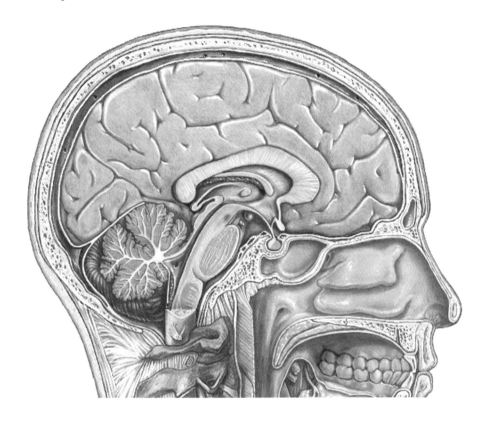

Draw your own lines and then label following features on the diagram.

   a. Dorsal root ganglion   **e.** Spinal nerve

   b. Pia mater   **f.** Dorsal horn

   c. Ventral root   **g.** Arachnoid mater

   d. Dura mater

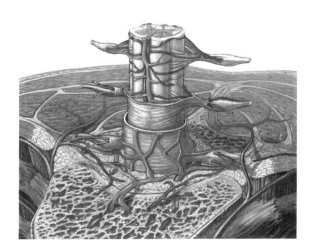

Fill in the Blank/Short Answer

1. The ventral horn of the spinal cord contains cell bodies of _____ neurons.

2. A raised ridge on the surface of the brain is known as a _____.

3. CSF is made from specialized capillaries known as _____.

4. The three components of the brainstem are the _____, _____, and _____.

5. The craniosacral division of the ANS is the _____ division.

6. Carpal tunnel syndrome is from entrapment of the _____ nerve.

7. The major nerve of the cervical plexus is the _____.

8. The sciatic nerve divides into the _____ and _____ nerves.

9. The nerve that innervates the extensor muscles of the upper limb is the _____.

10. The central nervous system is made up of the _____ and _____.

11. The peripheral nervous system consists of _____ pairs of cranial nerves and _____ pairs of spinal nerves.

12. The spinal cord terminates at the level of the _____ / _____ disc at the pointy structure known as the _____ _____.

13. The white matter of the cerebellum is known as the _____.

14. The passageway that connects the third and fourth ventricles is known as the _____.

Essay

1. List the 12 pairs of cranial nerves by name and Roman numeral, and indicate their function.

2. Trace the flow of cerebrospinal fluid beginning from the lateral ventricles of the brain.

3. Describe as many functions of the hypothalamus as possible.

Special Senses

4

LEARNING OBJECTIVES

Upon completion of this chapter, the student should be able to:

- Identify the external features of the eye
- Identify the three tunics of the eye and describe the structures found in each
- Describe the types of humors located within the internal chambers of the eye
- Identify the extraocular muscles of the eye and recall their cranial nerve innervation
- Differentiate between emmetropia, myopia, and hyperopia
- Identify the structures found in the external ear
- Identify the structures found in the middle ear
- Identify the structures found in the internal ear
- Identify the location of the receptors for hearing and equilibrium
- Locate the olfactory nerve and describe its relationship to the olfactory bulb, olfactory tract, and the receptors within the nasal mucosa
- Identify the gross features of the external tongue and describe the four primary tastes

SPECIAL SENSES OVERVIEW

The four classical special senses include sight, sound, smell, and taste. Some consider balance (equilibrium) as the fifth special sense since the receptors for balance are very specialized and localized to the inner ear. **Sight** is made possible by specialized photoreceptors located within the retina of the eye. **Hearing** (as well as equilibrium) is transmitted via the vibration of specialized mechanoreceptors located within the inner ear. Both smell (**olfaction**) and taste (**gustation**) are transmitted by chemoreceptors that respond to various chemicals dissolved in aqueous solution.

LAB ACTIVITY 4.1

External Features of the Eye

The majority of the eye is contained within, and protected by, the bony orbit of the skull. The external aspect of the eye is visible, however, through opened eyelids (palpebrae). Obvious structures in this view include the **sclera**, or white, of the eye; the **iris**, or colored part of the eye; the **pupil**, visualized as a black hole in the iris; and the **conjunctiva**, which externally may be seen on the undersurface of the eyelids.

For a unique interactive experience, click on the **3D Anatomy** *icon and then select* **3D Eye**.

3D Eye

From there you are able to manipulate a three-dimensional eye by rotating it, moving it, and zooming it in and out.

Identify and label the external features of the eye in the following figure.

CI Eye

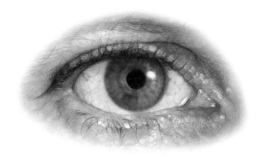

 LAB ACTIVITY 4.2

Layers (Tunics) of the Eye

The outermost tunic of the eye is referred to as the **fibrous tunic**. It consists of the thick, white **sclera** that makes up the majority of this layer. Anteriorly, the sclera ends and is replaced by the transparent **cornea**, which allows light to enter the eye. The middle layer is referred to as the **vascular tunic**. It consists primarily of the darkened **choroid**, which is made of vast layers of blood vessels that nourish the eye. Anteriorly is located the **ciliary body** consisting of the **ciliary muscle**, which attaches to the **lens** (via **suspensory ligaments**) to focus light on the retina, and the **ciliary processes**, which contain specialized capillaries responsible for secreting aqueous humor (to be discussed later). Also found in this layer is the pigmented **iris**, made up of layers of circular and radiating smooth muscle cells surrounding a central opening known as the **pupil**. The smooth muscle cells are under the control of the autonomic nervous system and contract or relax to regulate the amount of light entering the eye. The inner layer of the eye is known as the **neural (sensory) tunic,** and it is the location of the **retina**. The retina contains specialized **photoreceptors**, rods and cones, which are designed to respond to light. At the posterior aspect of the retina may be found the **optic disc**, or **blind spot**. The optic disc is void of neural receptors (hence the moniker, blind spot) and is the location where the optic nerve actually exits the eye.

Identify and label the three tunics of the eye and the features found in each in the following figure.

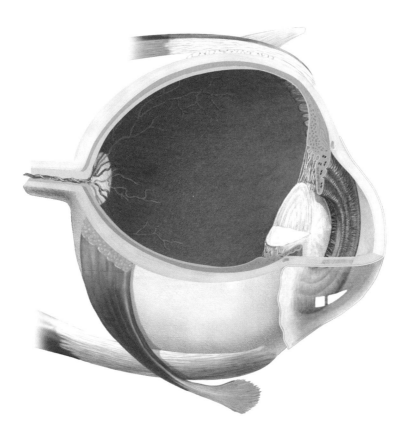

Located laterally to the optic disc is a small, yellowish, circular region known as the **macula lutea.** Within the macula is a smaller, central **fovea centralis**, which is the area of the eye with the greatest visual acuity. It contains the most densely packed region of cones in the retina.

To view an image of the macula lutea in AIA:
1. *Click on* **Clinical Illustrations**; *Select* "**All**," "**All**," "**All**," "**All**," *and* "**Ophthalmology**" *from the associated drop-down menus.*
2. *Click* "**Search**."
3. *Find the image titled* **Macula.**

CLINICAL APPLICATIONS

Human eyes are normally set for distant vision (20/20) when at rest. When light rays from an object 20 feet away reach the lens, the light is *refracted* (bent) so that the rays focus precisely on the retina. This "normal" vision is referred to as **emmetropia**. When viewing a close-up object, such as with reading, the lens must bulge (become more convex) in order to bend the light more sharply. The ability of the lens to change shape, that is, become either more concave or more convex, is called *accommodation*. **Farsightedness** (*hyperopia*) results when the lens cannot accommodate (bulge) appropriately or the eyeball is too short, causing the light rays to focus behind the retina leading to a blurred image. Farsighted individuals can still see distant images clearly, as it is easier for the lens to refract the more parallel light rays coming into the eye from a distance. A form of farsightedness resulting from a progressive loss in flexibility of the lens, commonly occurring after age 40, is known as **presbyopia** ("old eyes"). **Nearsightedness** (*myopia*) occurs when an individual is able to see objects right in front of them but cannot focus on images at a distance. In the case of myopia, the individual either has an eyeball that is too long or a lens that is too strong, causing the light rays to converge in front of the retina, again leading to a blurry image. In either case (myopia or hyperopia), corrective lenses (glasses or contact lenses) may be placed in front of the eye to refract the light rays before they enter the eye, causing the rays to focus precisely on the retina leading to clearer vision. Unequal curvature of either the lens or the cornea (a condition known as **astigmatism**) causes light rays to focus on multiple regions of the eye as lines rather than as a precise point, leading to a distorted image.

To view the following image in AIA:
1. *Click on Clinical Illustrations; Select "**Head and Neck**," "**All**," "**Medial**," "**Illustration**," and "**Optometry**" from the associated drop-down menus.*
2. *Click "**Search**."*
3. *Find the image titled **Normal, Near, and Farsightedness**.*

CI | Normal, Near, and Farsightedness

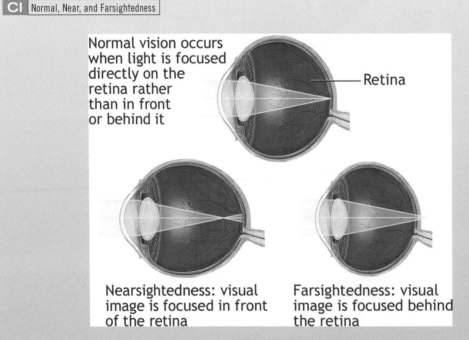

Normal vision occurs when light is focused directly on the retina rather than in front or behind it

Retina

Nearsightedness: visual image is focused in front of the retina

Farsightedness: visual image is focused behind the retina

LASIK (laser-assisted *in situ* keratomileusis) is a surgical procedure that uses lasers to actually reshape the cornea, bending the light before the hit reaches the lens and reducing or eliminating the need to wear corrective lenses (glasses or contacts).

To view images of the stages of the LASIK procedure in AIA:
1. *Click on Clinical Illustrations; Select "**Head and Neck**," "**All**," "**Anterior**," "**Illustration**," and "**Optometry**" from the associated drop-down menus.*
2. *Click "**Search**."*
3. *Find the associated images.*

LAB ACTIVITY 4.3

The Internal Eye

Internally, the lens divides the eye into two fluid-filled compartments: the anterior segment and the posterior segment. The **posterior segment** is filled with a jelly-like fluid known as **vitreous humor**. The vitreous humor reinforces the eyeball and helps to maintain its shape. The vitreous humor is stagnant; that is, it is not continually replenished or replaced once it is initially formed. The **anterior segment** of the eye, by contrast, is filled with a water-like **aqueous humor**. The aqueous humor is continually produced by specialized capillaries within the ciliary processes and is subsequently drained via the canal of Schlemm and recirculated to venous circulation. Continuous production of the aqueous humor provides nutrients for some internal eye structures such as the avascular lens and cornea and also helps to maintain the intraocular pressure of the eye.

Compare and label the lens along with the segments of the eye and the ciliary body in the following figure and illustration.

 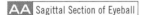

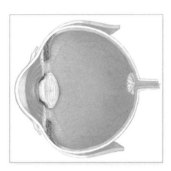 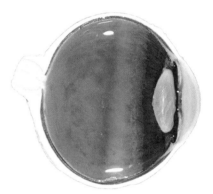

CLINICAL APPLICATIONS

An overproduction of aqueous humor or the inability to drain excess fluid can lead to an increase in intraocular pressure known as **glaucoma**. Glaucoma is often asymptomatic until advanced stages, presenting with a gradual loss of vision but can sometimes present with eye pain. Glaucoma is more common in the elderly and can eventually lead to blindness as a result of damage to the optic nerve.

To view an image of glaucoma in AIA:
1. *Click on Clinical Illustrations; Select "**Head and Neck**," "**All**," "**Non-standard**," "**Illustration**," and "**Ophthalmology**" from the associated drop-down menus.*
2. *Click "**Search**."*
3. *Find the image titled **Glaucoma**.*

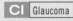

Another common eye condition associated with aging is a **cataract**. The lens of the eye is made primarily of crystalline proteins that are transparent in the young but become increasingly stiff and somewhat opaque as we age. This causes the lens to get cloudy, leading to a progressive loss of vision. Cataracts can lead to blurry vision, difficulty driving at night, and an increase in glares from bright lights.

To view an image of a cataract in AIA:
1. *Click on Clinical Illustrations; Select "**Head and Neck**," "**All**," "**Anterior**," "**Illustration**," and "**Ophthalmology**" from the associated drop-down menus.*
2. *Click "**Search**."*
3. *Find the image titled **Cataract**.*

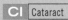

LAB ACTIVITY 4.4

Extrinsic Eye Muscles

There are six extrinsic eye muscles that attach to the outside of the eyeball allowing for voluntary movement of the eye. The cranial nerve innervation was discussed in the nervous system chapter but will be revisited here. There are four rectus (rectus: straight) muscles that attach to the eye. They are the **superior rectus**, **inferior rectus**, **medial rectus**, and **lateral rectu**s. The **superior oblique** muscle has the same origin as the four rectus muscles, but then its tendon wraps around the small trochlea (trochlea: pulley) to attach obliquely on the superior aspect of the eye. Contraction of this muscle then will cause the eye to look down and out. Lastly, the **inferior oblique** originates from the medial aspect of the orbital floor and then attaches obliquely to the inferior surface of the lateral eye. Contraction of this muscle causes the eye to look up and out. The superior oblique is innervated by the ***trochlear nerve*** (CN IV), the lateral rectus by the ***abducens nerve*** (CN VI), and the remaining four muscles are all under the control of the ***oculomotor nerve*** (CN III).

Compare and label the extraocular eye muscles from the lateral aspect in the following illustration and cadaver photo. To view a similar image, you may go to

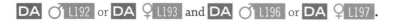

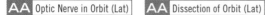

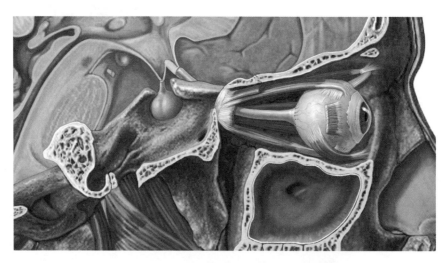

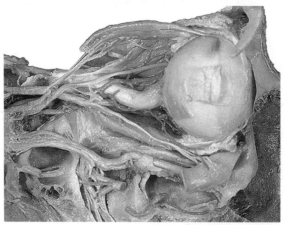

Now compare and label the extraocular eye muscles from the anterior aspect in the following illustration and cadaver photo. To view a similar image, you may go to

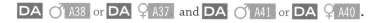

| AA | Extrinsic Eye Muscles (Ant) | | AA | Eyeball & Extrinsic Eye Muscles |

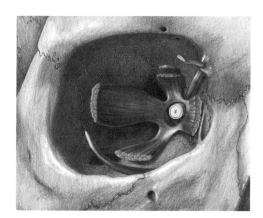 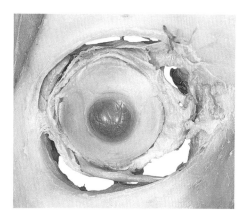

LAB ACTIVITY 4.5

Anatomy of the Ear

The ear houses the sensory receptors for hearing as well equilibrium (balance). Both senses rely on the movement of fluid over specialized **_mechanoreceptors_** containing special, hair-like cilia for excitation. Anatomically, the ear is divided into three sections: the outer ear, middle ear, and inner ear.

For a unique interactive experience, click on the **3D Anatomy** _icon and then select_ **3D Ear**.

| 3D | Ear |

From there you are able to manipulate a three-dimensional ear by rotating it, moving it, and zooming it in and out.

The **external ear** consists of the **auricle (pinna)** and **external auditory (acoustic) canal (meatus)**, stopping at the **tympanic membrane** (eardrum). Lining the external acoustic canal are found ceruminous glands producing sticky **_cerumen_**, which is thought to repel insects from taking up residence in your ears. The **middle ear**, separated from the external ear by the tympanic membrane, consists of three small bones collectively known as **ossicles**. The three ossicles are the **malleus** (hammer), **incus** (anvil), and **stapes** (stirrup). Sound waves vibrating against the tympanic membrane are amplified by the vibration of the three ossicles, which then send the sound waves on to the inner ear. Also located in the middle ear is the opening of one end of the **pharyngotympanic (auditory, eustachian) tube**. The other end, as the name suggests, opens into the pharynx—specifically into the posterior aspect of the nasopharynx. This tube is normally collapsed but serves to equilibrate air pressure in the middle ear cavity so it equals atmospheric air pressure in the external ear. This equality in pressure allows for optimum vibration of the tympanic membrane. If you have ever had the experience of your ears "popping," say in an airplane, while yawning, or when climbing a mountain in your car, you have seen the difference in your lack of ability to hear acutely with "clogged ears." This intimate connection between the pharynx (throat) and the middle ear cavity is why it is fairly common for toddlers with immature immune systems to associate middle ear infections (otitis media) with sore throats.

CLINICAL APPLICATIONS

On occasion, some children may develop an accumulation of fluid in the middle ear resulting from recurring bouts of otitis media. In severe cases, this fluid buildup can lead to a loss of hearing and perhaps even affect speech development. Ear tubes (tympanostomy tubes) are small tubes inserted into the tympanic membrane via a tiny incision, allowing for drainage of the middle ear and an equalization of pressure. The tubes will then typically fall out on their own as the child grows, allowing the holes to heal shut on their own.

To view an image of ear tubes in AIA:
1. *Click on Clinical Illustrations; Select "**Head and Neck**," "**All**," "**Non-standard**," "**Illustration**," and "**Pediatrics**" from the associated drop-down menus.*
2. *Click "**Search**."*
3. *Find the image titled **Ear Tube Insertion**.*

CI | Ear Tube Insertion

The **inner ear** houses the sensory receptors for both hearing and equilibrium. The **vestibule** is found just opposite of the oval window, which is where the stapes attaches from the other side. It houses the receptors for **static balance**, which is balance when you are still. These receptors, called **maculae**, respond to changes in the pull of gravity on the head. The **semicircular canals**, as the name suggests, are three fluid-filled canals that are aligned along three distinct planes. This allows them to respond to **angular movement (dynamic balance)** regardless of the direction. The receptors located here, the **crista ampullaris**, respond to the movement of fluid as your head is in motion. The receptors for hearing, the **spiral organ of Corti**, are found within the snail shell–looking apparatus known as the **cochlea**. Sound vibrations transmitted to the inner ear fluids from the ossicles allow for the stimulation of these specialized receptors. Nerve impulses for both hearing and balance are transmitted along the **vestibulocochlear nerve** (CN VIII).

To observe an animated overview of the mechanism of hearing:
1. *Click on **Clinical Animations**; Select "**Head and Neck**," "**All**," and "**Otolaryngology (ENT)**" from the associated drop-down menus.*
2. *Click "**Search**."*
3. *Find the animation titled **Hearing and the Cochlea**.*

→ | Hearing and the Cochlea

Identify and label the three regions of the ear and the major features found in each using the following figure.

CI Ear Anatomy

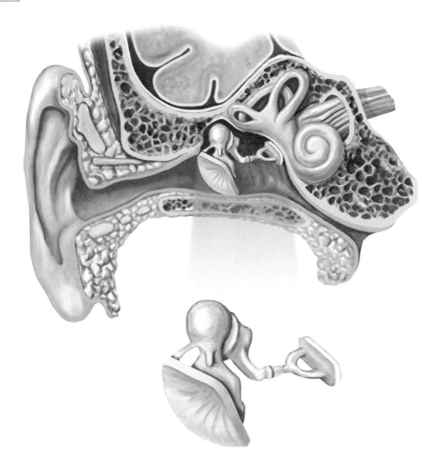

Identify and label some common features of the external ear such as the pinna, lobule, and external acoustic meatus in the following figure.

AA Auricle of Ear

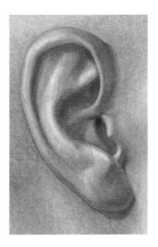

Identify and label some common features of the middle ear such as the tympanic membrane, malleus, incus, and stapes in the following figure.

CI Eardrum (Tympanic Membrane) Anatomy

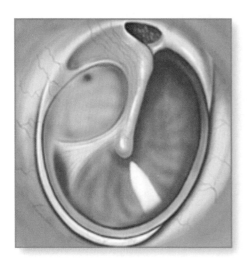 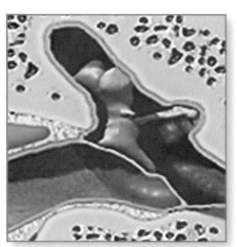

Identify and label some common features of the inner ear such as the cochlea, the semicircular canals, and the vestibular and cochlear branches of CN VIII in the following figure.

AA External, Middle, & Internal Ear

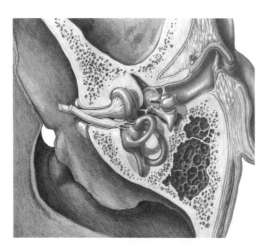

LAB ACTIVITY 4.6

The Sense of Smell

The receptors for smell (**olfaction**) are actually **_chemoreceptors_** whose nerve endings are found in the roof of the nasal cavity, protected by a thin layer of mucus. In order to stimulate these receptors, an airborne chemical must dissolve through the mucus and bind to these chemoreceptors. The axons from these thousands of receptors bundle into multiple olfactory filaments that comprise the **_olfactory nerve_** (CN I). These filaments leave the nasal cavity and enter into the cranial cavity through many small holes (the cribriform plate) in the ethmoid bone. From here, the fibers synapse in the olfactory bulb that lies along the top of the cribriform plate and then proceed via the olfactory tract to the sensory cortex of the brain for interpretation. Because smell is dependent on chemicals dissolving through the mucus layer on the nasal cavity, it is easy to see why it is harder to smell when one is suffering with a condition such as the common cold. The excess mucus production becomes too thick for the airborne chemicals to dissolve through, leading to a decreased ability to distinguish smells.

Identify and label some common features of the nasal cavity such as the olfactory bulb, cribriform plate, nasal conchae, and nasal mucosa in the following figure. To view a similar image with a close-up of the olfactory bulb and receptor cells, you may go to **CI** | Sense of Smell | _to view an image labeled Sense of smell._

AA | Olfactory Nerve in Nasal Cavity

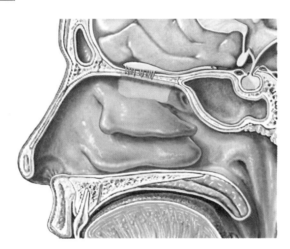

LAB ACTIVITY 4.7

The Sense of Taste

The receptors for taste (**gustation**) are actually **chemoreceptors** whose nerve endings are found in taste buds along the sides of bumps of the tongue called **papillae**, protected by a thin layer of saliva. In order to stimulate these receptors, a chemical must dissolve through the saliva and bind to these chemoreceptors. Not all papillae contain taste buds, however. The approximately 10 to 12 **circumvallate papillae** separate the anterior two-thirds of the tongue from the posterior one-third of the tongue and do contain receptors for taste. **Foliate papillae** are grouped into two small regions found laterally along the tongue and contain taste buds as well. The more numerous **fungiform papillae** also contain taste buds and may be found throughout the surface of the tongue. The **filiform papillae**, however, do not contain taste buds. They are there to provide friction on the surface of the tongue to help position food and offer protection to the surface of the tongue. Animals that groom themselves with their tongue, such as cats, have very well-developed filiform papillae that may cause a lick from them to feel very rough and scratchy.

The four common tastes include sweet, salty, sour, and bitter. Although receptors for each of these may be found throughout the tongue, there seem to be areas of the tongue that are more sensitive to one taste more than another. **Sweet** and **salty** receptors tend to be focused more to the anterior of the tongue. With sweet (glucose or sugar) being the primary source of energy for the body, and salty (sodium chloride) having the extremely important roles of maintaining the resting cell membrane potentials, initiating nerve impulse generation and muscle contraction, to name a few, it seems appropriate that these receptors are to the front of the tongue as we introduce new foods to the mouth to be tasted. **Bitter** receptors are the most sensitive of all taste receptors and may be stimulated with the lowest concentration of chemical stimulus. The bitter receptors are located at the back of the tongue. It is thought that this may be an innate safety mechanism since, in nature, many natural toxins and even many spoiled foods have a bitter taste. Because virtually everything that is ingested must pass by these bitter receptors, stimulation of these receptors may cause the person to spit out the potential toxin before swallowing it into the body. **Sour** receptors are typically clustered more along the sides of the tongue and respond to many types of acidic foods. A more recently discovered fifth taste, called **umami**, responds to the amino acid glutamate that is described as a savory or meaty taste.

Identify and label some common features of the tongue including the four types of papillae in the following figure.

AA | Surface of Tongue (Dorsal)

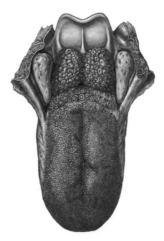

SPECIAL SENSES REVIEW EXERCISES

Matching

_____	**1.**	Retina
_____	**2.**	Iris
_____	**3.**	Ciliary body
_____	**4.**	Cornea
_____	**5.**	Fovea centralis
_____	**6.**	Choroid
_____	**7.**	Optic disc
_____	**8.**	Sclera

a. vascular tunic
b. sensory tunic
c. fibrous tunic

Matching

_____	**1.**	Malleus
_____	**2.**	Pinna
_____	**3.**	Cochlea
_____	**4.**	Lobule
_____	**5.**	Semicircular canals
_____	**6.**	External auditory canal
_____	**7.**	Stapes
_____	**8.**	Vestibule
_____	**9.**	Incus

a. external ear
b. inner ear
c. middle ear

Labeling

Draw your own lines and then label the following features on the diagram.

a. Lens
b. Cornea
c. Inferior oblique
d. Optic nerve
e. Superior rectus
f. Sclera
g. Retina
h. Inferior rectus
i. Iris

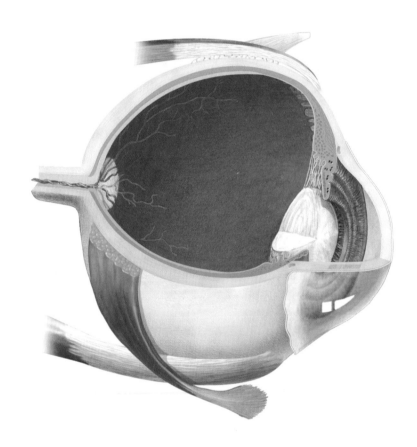

Draw your own lines and then label the following features on the diagram.

a. Semicircular canals   f. Stapes

b. Pinna   g. Tympanic membrane

c. Malleus   h. Lobule

d. Cochlea   i. Incus

e. External auditory canal   j. Vestibulocochlear nerve

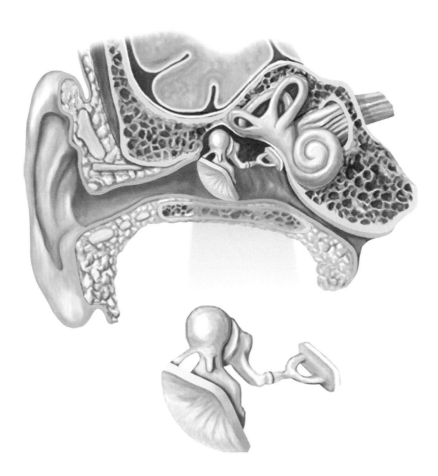

Fill in the Blank/Short Answer

1. The colored portion of the eye is known as the _____.

2. The two types of photoreceptors found in the retina are the _____ and

    _____.

3. The "blind spot" is more properly known as the _____.

4. The muscle that causes the eye to look down and out is the _____.

5. The _____ nerve innervates the lateral rectus.

6. Bulging of the lens to focus the eyes is known as _____.

7. Cloudiness of the lens that is more common in the aged is known as _____.

8. _____ humor is continually produced and reabsorbed within the anterior segment

    of the eye.

9. At rest, the lens of the eye is normally set for _____ vision.

10. The "ear drum" is more properly known as the _____ _____.

11. The vestibule has receptors called maculae for _____ balance while the semicircular

    canals contain receptors called crista ampullaris for _____ balance.

12. A middle ear infection is also known as _____ _____.

13. The waxy substance secreted into the external auditory canal is called _____

14. Filaments of the olfactory nerve pass from the nasal cavity into the cranium through the

    _____ of the ethmoid bone.

15. Taste and smell are detected by specialized receptors known as _____.

16. The _____ papillae do not contain any taste buds.

17. The most sensitive of all taste receptors respond to the taste of _____ and are

    located at the back of the tongue.

Essay

1. Describe the pathway of light through the eye (include all transparent structures that the light will
    pass through) until it reaches the photoreceptors of the retina.

2. Discuss the differences between emmetropia, myopia, and hyperopia.

3. Describe the pathway of sound waves as they travel from the air into the cochlea.

Endocrine System

LEARNING OBJECTIVES

Upon completion of this chapter, the student should be able to:

- Locate the hypothalamus and provide examples of functions of its major hormones

- Locate the pituitary gland and provide examples of functions of its major hormones, distinguishing between those of the adenohypophysis and neurohypophysis

- Locate the pineal gland and provide examples of functions of its major hormones

- Locate the thyroid gland and provide examples of functions of its major hormones

- Locate the parathyroid gland and provide examples of functions of its major hormones

- Locate the pancreas and provide examples of functions of its major hormones, distinguishing between endocrine and exocrine secretions

- Locate the adrenal gland and provide examples of functions of its major hormones, distinguishing between cortical and medullary secretions

- Locate the male testis and provide examples of functions of its major hormones

- Locate the female ovary and provide examples of functions of its major hormones

ENDOCRINE SYSTEM OVERVIEW

The endocrine system is the second major organ system involved in the maintenance of homeostasis, along with the nervous system. Because of the intimate relationship between the nervous and the endocrine systems, some scholars study both systems collectively as the "neuroendocrine" system. While the nervous system is the "fast-acting" system that controls and coordinates via nerve impulses, the endocrine system is the "slow-acting" system that exerts its control via chemical secretions known as **hormones**. As hormones are produced, they are secreted directly into the bloodstream and then travel, via the cardiovascular system, to the specific receptors found on the target tissues (effectors) of the body. Glands that are exocrine in nature do not secrete their product into circulation. Exocrine glands expel their secretions via a duct that will open into a hollow organ or onto the surface of the body. To make matters more confusing, some of the glands we will explore in this chapter will be uniquely endocrine while other glands will have a dual role producing both endocrine and exocrine secretions. Additionally, we sometimes find organs that are not typically considered "endocrine" in nature, such as the skin, duodenum, or the heart, that have hormone-producing cells within them.

To observe an animated overview of the endocrine system:
*1. Click on **Clinical Animations**; Select "**All**," "**Endocrine**," and "**All**" from the associated drop-down menus.*
*2. Click "**Search**."*
*3. Find the animation titled **Endocrine Glands-General Overview.***

➡ Endocrine Glands—General Overview

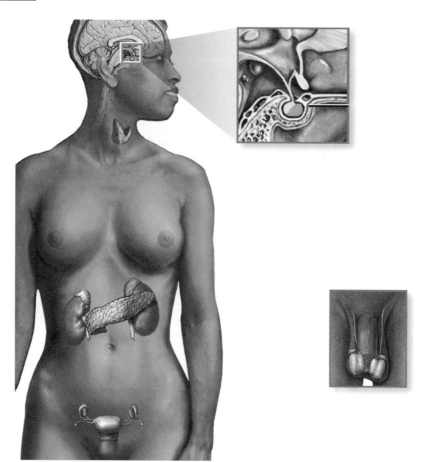

LAB ACTIVITY 5.1

Hypothalamus

The **hypothalamus** is a neuroendocrine structure found within the diencephalon of the brain (along with the thalamus and epithalamus). While the hypothalamus is responsible for regulating a wide array of visceral functions, its influence over the pituitary gland will be considered here. The hypothalamus synthesizes a number of regulating hormones that then exert their effect on the anterior pituitary gland. These hormones can be either stimulatory (***releasing hormones***) or inhibitory (***inhibiting hormones***). In addition, the hypothalamus produces two major hormones (***oxytocin*** and ***antidiuretic hormone***) that are then stored in, and ultimately secreted by, the posterior pituitary gland.

CI Hypothalamus Hormone Production

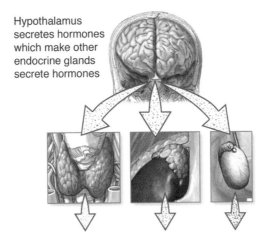

Hypothalamus secretes hormones which make other endocrine glands secrete hormones

EPITHALAMUS

The **epithalamus** is also found in the diencephalon of the brain and contains the **pineal gland (pineal body)** suspended posteriorly from its roof. While little is known about the function of the pineal gland, it is associated with the production of ***melatonin***. Melatonin is a hormone most recognized for its role in helping to maintain circadian rhythms and regulating sleep/wake cycles. It also appears to exhibit some effect over the timing and release of female reproductive hormones.

PITUITARY GLAND

The **pituitary gland (hypophysis cerebri)** is a small, pea-like structure that may be found connected superiorly to the hypothalamus via the infundibulum and nestled within the sella turcica of the sphenoid bone. The pituitary gland is often referred to as the "master gland" because of the widespread effects its hormones exert on the body. The pituitary gland actually has two distinctly different functional regions, the **anterior pituitary** and the **posterior pituitary**, which will be discussed separately.

Anterior Pituitary

The **anterior pituitary (adenohypophysis)** consists of glandular tissue and is responsible for both the manufacturing and the secretion of its hormones. While the anterior pituitary produces its own hormones, it does so at the direction of the releasing and inhibiting hormones from the hypothalamus. As many as seven different hormones are known to be secreted by the anterior pituitary, and of those, four are considered to be **"tropic"** hormones. Tropic hormones are those stimulatory hormones that bind to other endocrine glands, thereby causing those glands to secrete more of their respective hormones. The four tropic hormones secreted by the anterior pituitary include ***thyroid-stimulating hormone (TSH or thyrotropin)***, which influences the activity of the thyroid gland; ***adrenocorticotropic hormone (ACTH or corticotropin)***, which influences the activity of the adrenal cortex; ***follicle-stimulating hormone (FSH)***, which guides gamete production in both males and females; and ***luteinizing hormone (LH)***, which regulates hormone production in the gonads of both sexes. Some consider all hormones of the adenohypophysis as tropic because they are all stimulatory in some fashion, although the remaining hormones do not act on endocrine glands proper. The remaining hormones of the anterior pituitary are ***growth hormone (GH, somatotropin, or somatotropic hormone [STH])***, which exerts most of its effects on skeletal and muscular growth; ***prolactin (PRL or mammotropin)***, which is responsible for the production of milk in the lactating mother; and ***melanocyte-stimulating hormone (MSH or melanotropin)***, which stimulates the melanocytes of the epidermis to release the pigment melanin, thereby affecting skin and hair tones.

Posterior Pituitary

The **posterior pituitary (neurohypophysis)** is made of nervous tissue and is not capable of manufacturing its own hormones. Instead, it stores two hormones that have been made by the hypothalamus. The posterior pituitary is actually directly connected to the hypothalamus by a thin stalk known as the **infundibulum**. Nerve impulses from the hypothalamus travel down the infundibulum and trigger the release of the two stored hormones as needed. ***Oxytocin*** is a hormone that is responsible for the powerful uterine contractions associated with childbirth. Once the baby is born, oxytocin continues to be a hormone of importance for the lactating mother as oxytocin is responsible for the ejection, or let-down, of milk during breast-feeding. Both of these instances of oxytocin release are rather rare examples of positive feedback mechanisms in the body. ***Antidiuretic hormone (ADH)*** is responsible for inhibiting urine production. "Diuresis" is the term for an increased production of urine. ADH, by contrast, is a hormone that reduces the amount of urine produced at the kidneys, thereby allowing for blood volume and blood pressure to increase. ADH may also be referred to as ***vasopressin*** because of its ability to cause vasoconstriction in smaller blood vessels, also leading to an increase in blood pressure. Alcohol and caffeine are two known substances that interfere with the ability of ADH to regulate urine production, causing diuresis and possible dehydration.

Identify and label the two divisions of the pituitary gland in the following figure. Also find the pineal gland, the hypothalamus, and the infundibulum.

To locate the image in AIA:

1. *Click on **Atlas Anatomy**; Select "**Head and Neck**," "**Endocrine**," "**Medial**," and "**Illustration**" from the associated drop-down menus.*
2. *Click "**Search**."*
3. *Find the image titled **Sagittal Section of Brain**.*

AA | Sagittal Section of Brain

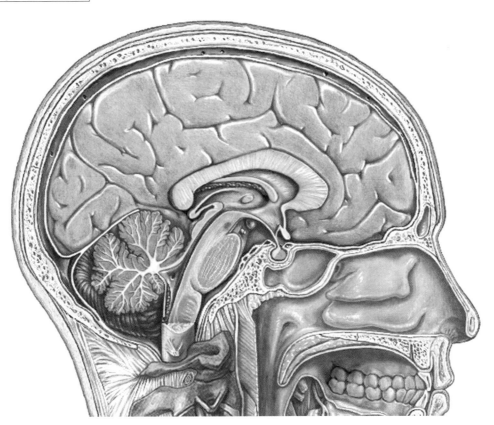

CLINICAL APPLICATIONS

Diabetes insipidus (DI; *diabetes*: to pass through—as with urination; *insipidus*: lack of taste) is a condition associated with a hyposecretion of ADH from the neurohypophysis. In the absence of ADH, excessive urination (**diuresis**) results. Generally DI is not too major of an issue if the patient's thirst response is functional. Diuresis will lead to an excessive thirst (**polydipsia**) causing an increase in fluid ingestion, which will then compensate for the condition. In cases of the unconscious patient or one without an intact thirst response, it is important to regulate fluid intake to help maintain homeostasis.

LAB ACTIVITY 5.2

Thyroid Gland

The **thyroid gland** is a somewhat butterfly-shaped gland located just inferior to the thyroid cartilage (Adam's apple) that secretes two major hormones. **_Thyroid hormone (TH)_** is the body's main hormone of metabolism and comes in two forms: T4 (thyroxine or tetraiodothyronine) and T3 (triiodothyronine). Thyroid hormone is produced by follicular cells, which surround colloid-filled follicles. This **colloid** is a precursor to thyroid hormone, which cannot be completely synthesized in the absence of iodine. If someone's diet is deficient in iodine, the follicles accumulate colloid, and the entire gland enlarges forming what is referred to as a colloidal **goiter**. Between the follicles of the gland are found clusters of cells referred to as parafollicular, or C cells. The parafollicular cells are responsible for the secretion of **_calcitonin_**. Calcitonin is antagonistic to parathyroid hormone and is released in response to high blood calcium levels (hypercalcemia), stimulating the deposition of calcium in bone.

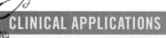 **CLINICAL APPLICATIONS**

Diseases of the thyroid gland are among the most common endocrine disorders. An overactive thyroid gland (**hyperthyroidism**) leads to an increase in the body's metabolism, associated with an unexplained weight loss, nervousness, anxiety, difficulty concentrating, and a sensitivity to heat. Common causes of an overactive thyroid include Graves disease, inflammation of the thyroid (**_thyroiditis_**), and both cancerous and noncancerous growths. Hyperthyroidism is usually treatable with medications and even surgery and is rarely life threatening. **Hypothyroidism**, where the thyroid gland is not active enough, is a much more common condition. With hypothyroidism, there is a decrease in the body's metabolism leading to unexplained weight gain, fatigue, weakness, and depression. The most common cause of hypothyroidism is inflammation of the thyroid gland, which damages the gland's cells. An enlarged thyroid gland may often be diagnosed via a **_thyroid ultrasound_**, which uses high-frequency sound waves to make a picture of the gland. Treatments for an overactive thyroid such as surgery to remove part of the gland can also cause hypothyroidism. The purpose of hypothyroidism treatment is to replace the thyroid hormone that is lacking. Generally speaking, lifelong therapy is required and thyroid hormone levels should be checked on a periodic basis, regardless of the presence or absence of symptoms.

To view some images of hypothyroidism and hyperthyroidism in AIA:
1. _Click on Clinical Illustrations; Select "**Head and Neck**," "**Endocrine**," "**All**," "**All**," and "**Endocrinology**" from the associated drop-down menus._
2. _Click "**Search**."_
3. _Find the corresponding images._

PARATHYROID GLANDS

The **parathyroid glands** are found on the posterior aspect of the thyroid gland and usually consist of four BB-sized glands (two on each side). The parathyroid glands secrete **_parathyroid hormone (PTH)_**, which is considered to be the most important hormone for regulating blood calcium levels. PTH is released in response to low blood calcium levels (hypocalcemia) and functions as an antagonist to calcitonin. PTH causes calcium to be released from bone, enhances reabsorption of calcium by the kidney, and increases calcium absorption from the intestines.

● *Identify and label the thyroid and parathyroid glands in the following figures.*
To locate the image in AIA:
1. *Click on **Atlas Anatomy**; Select "**Head and Neck**," "**Endocrine**," "**Lateral**," and "**Illustration**" from the associated drop-down menus.*
2. *Click "**Search**."*
3. *Find the image titled **Glands of Head & Neck (Lat)**.*

AA Glands of Head & Neck (Lat)

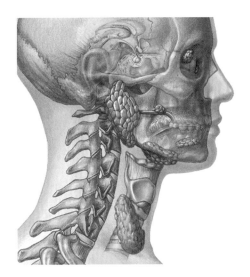

● 1. *Click on **Clinical Illustrations**; Select "**Head and Neck**," "**Endocrine**," "**Anterior**," "**Illustration**," and "Endocrinology" from the associated drop-down menus.*
2. *Click "**Search**."*
3. *Find the image titled **Parathyroid glands**.*

CI Parathyroid Glands

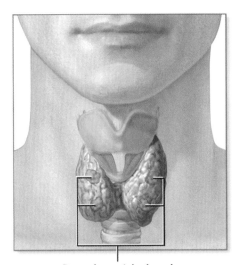

Parathyroid glands

To view a similar image of the thyroid gland, you may go to **DA** ♂ A78 *or* **DA** ♀ A77.

LAB ACTIVITY 5.3

Thymus Gland

The **thymus** gland is located in the superior mediastinum (thorax) just posterior to the sternum but anterior to the heart. The thymus is an important gland of the lymphatic (immune) system and secretes *thymosin*, which has the role of T-lymphocyte maturation. T lymphocytes are responsible for cell-mediated immunity, rejection of foreign tissue, and the recognition of virus-infected cells as well as cancer cells. The thymus is prominent at birth, reaches maximum function during childhood, and then begins to atrophy at adolescence. By adulthood, as it becomes invested with connective tissue, the thymus retains only rudimentary function.

Identify and label the thymus in the following figure. To view the image in AIA, go to

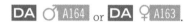

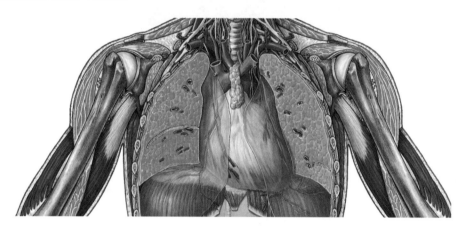

LAB ACTIVITY 5.4

Pancreas

The **pancreas** is a long slender organ located in the abdominal cavity just posterior to the stomach. It is a mixed organ in that it contains **exocrine** cells (*acinar* cells) responsible for producing digestive enzymes and **endocrine** cells (*islet* cells) responsible for secreting hormones. *Insulin* is a hormone that is released by the islet cells in response to high blood sugar levels (hyperglycemia). *Glucagon*, also secreted by the islet cells, is antagonistic to insulin and acts primarily on the liver to increase blood sugar levels when they get too low.

Identify and label the pancreas in the following figure. To view the image in AIA, go to

 ♂ A214 or ♀ A211 .

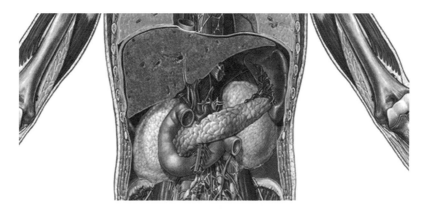

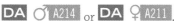 **CLINICAL APPLICATIONS**

Diabetes mellitus (diabetes: to pass through—as with urination; mellitus: honey, sweetness) is a condition typically associated with a hyposecretion of insulin from the pancreas or from a lack of sensitivity of body cells to circulating insulin. While blood glucose is available in circulation, the body cells do not have access to them as fuel. As a result, blood glucose levels rise above normal (hyperglycemia) and then spill over into the urine; hence, the term "sweet urine." Since the body cells cannot use available glucose, stored proteins and fats are broken down for fuel resulting in the accumulation of ketone bodies. As ketone levels rise, the pH of the blood declines leading to a very severe condition known as diabetic ketoacidosis (DKA), which can be fatal if untreated. Diabetes mellitus is recognized by three cardinal signs sometimes referred to as the "3 P's"—**polyuria** (excessive urination), **polydipsia** (excessive thirst), and **polyphagia** (excessive hunger). Type 2 diabetes mellitus is the most common form of the disease and is also known as adult-onset diabetes or **NIDDM** (non–insulin-dependent diabetes mellitus) since some patients can control the condition through diet and exercise. Type 1 diabetes mellitus is known as juvenile diabetes or **IDDM** (insulin-dependent diabetes mellitus) and is an autoimmune disease where the immune system attacks certain pancreatic islet cells. As a result, patients with type 1 diabetes must take insulin in order to survive. **Gestational diabetes** is a condition that occurs in pregnant women who otherwise do not present with signs and symptoms of diabetes mellitus. Gestational diabetes generally resolves on its own following the birth of the baby.

To view some images of diabetes causes and related treatments in AIA:
1. *Click on Clinical Illustrations; Select "**All**," "**Endocrine**," "**All**," "**All**," and "**Endocrinology**" from the associated drop-down menus.*
2. *Click "**Search**."*
3. *Find the corresponding images.*

ADRENAL GLANDS

The two **adrenal (suprarenal) glands** are sometimes referred to as our "stress glands" and may be found resting upon the top of each kidney. Each gland is actually like two glands in one with the central adrenal medulla and the peripheral adrenal cortex having distinct functions. The **medulla** is derived from neural tissue and is under the direct influence of the sympathetic nervous system, providing for the "fight-or-flight" response associated with acute stressors. It is responsible for the secretion of epinephrine (adrenaline) and norepinephrine (noradrenaline). The **cortex** is glandular in nature and is actually made up of three layers (zonas) of cells. The outer zona glomerulosa secretes **mineralocorticoids** (primarily **aldosterone**), which help regulate water and electrolyte balance (mainly sodium); the middle zona fasciculata secretes **glucocorticoids** (primarily **cortisone** and **cortisol**), which help the body resist chronic stressors; and the inner zona reticularis secretes **sex hormones** in small amounts. These sex hormones likely do not have much effect during our reproductive years but may become more important with age as the reproductive organs themselves slow down in function.

Identify and label the adrenal glands in the following figure. To view the image in AIA, go to

DA ♂ A232 or DA ♀ A231 .

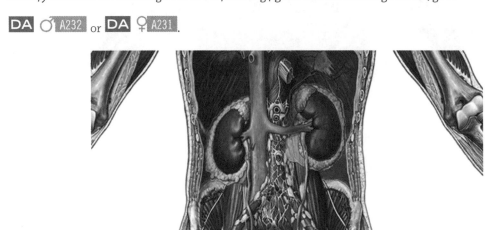

THE GONADS

The male and female **gonads** are part of the reproductive system and each produce both **gametes** (sex cells) and sex hormones.

Testes

The **testes** (male gonads) are paired organs suspended from the pelvis in a thin sac known as the scrotum. In addition to the production of **sperm** (sex cells), the testes are primarily responsible for the production of testosterone. **Testosterone** is an androgen (male hormone) responsible for the growth and maturation of the male reproductive system as well as causing an increase in libido, or sex drive. Testosterone production increases at puberty and is responsible for the secondary sex characteristics seen in men such as deepening of the voice, distribution of facial and pubic hair, and muscle and bone development.

Identify and label the testes in the following figure. To view the image in AIA, go to

AA Male Pelvic Organs (Ant)

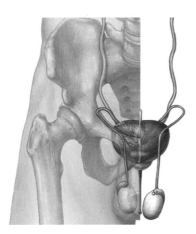

Ovaries

The **ovaries** (female gonads) are paired organs located in the pelvic cavity just lateral to the uterus. In addition to the development of **ova** (sex cells), the ovaries are primarily responsible for the production of **estrogen** and **progesterone** beginning at puberty. Estrogen is responsible for the secondary sex characteristics seen in women such as maturation of the reproductive organs, distribution of pubic hair, and breast development. Progesterone, together with estrogen, is responsible for the cyclic (monthly) changes in the uterus in preparation for pregnancy—the menstrual, or uterine, cycle. With conception, progesterone levels stay elevated until implantation of the embryo occurs and the developing placenta can assume the role of regulating the pregnancy.

Identify and label the ovaries in the following figure. To view the image in AIA, go to

AA Female Pelvic Organs (Ant)

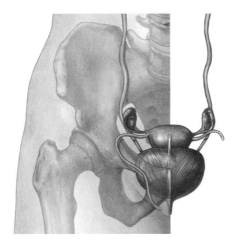

CLINICAL APPLICATIONS

Dysmenorrhea, an uncomfortable and sometimes painful menstrual period, is the most commonly reported menstrual disorder. More than half of all menstruating women are thought to have pain for at least 1 to 2 days/month. Primary dysmenorrhea is the pain commonly referred to as "menstrual cramps." Pain usually occurs just before the onset of menstruation and then decreases throughout the duration of the period as the lining of the uterus is shed. Primary dysmenorrhea will often begin soon after a girl starts having menstrual periods. In many women, menstruation becomes less painful with age and symptoms often improve after the birth of a child. Secondary dysmenorrhea tends to appear later in life and is the result of some other reproductive disorder. In contrast to primary dysmenorrhea, the secondary variety tends to get worse with age rather than better. Secondary dysmenorrhea may be caused by such conditions as endometriosis, fibroids, or sometimes adhesions from scar tissue resulting from prior surgeries or infections. Dysmenorrhea is often treated with pain medication or a form of the birth control pill to help regulate the menstrual cycle. Remember though—while we are dealing with a reproductive system condition—it is indeed a condition under the direct control of the endocrine system. While the actual pain may be associated with actions of the uterus, the uterus is just doing what hormones from the ovaries tell it to do. Of course, the ovaries are likewise doing what hormones from the adenohypophysis are telling them to do, and the adenohypophysis is simply acting on behalf of hormones secreted by the hypothalamus. While the glands of the endocrine system are not as large and impressive as organs in some other systems, a small change in hormone secretion by a single gland can have widespread effects on the body's ability to maintain homeostasis.

To view some images of hormones and glands involved in the menstrual cycle in AIA:

1. *Click on Clinical Illustrations; Select "**All**," "**Reproductive**," "**All**," "**All**," and "**Endocrinology**" from the associated drop-down menus.*
2. *Click "**Search**."*
3. *Find the corresponding images.*

ENDOCRINE SYSTEM REVIEW EXERCISES

Matching

_____ **1.** Adrenal gland

_____ **2.** Pituitary gland

_____ **3.** Testes

_____ **4.** Thymus

_____ **5.** Parathyroid gland

_____ **6.** Hypothalamus

_____ **7.** Pancreas

_____ **8.** Ovaries

_____ **9.** Thyroid gland

_____ **10.** Pineal gland

a. suspended from the roof of the diencephalon

b. in the superior mediastinum, anterior to the heart

c. located the pelvic cavity

d. located in the abdomen, posterior to the stomach

e. found in the diencephalon, attached to the neurohypophysis via the infundibulum

f. butterfly-shaped organ in the neck

g. found atop of the kidneys

h. found suspended from the pelvis in the scrotum

i. 4 BB-sized organs found in the neck

j. found in the sella turcica of the sphenoid bone

Matching

_____ **1.** Adrenal gland

_____ **2.** Pituitary gland

_____ **3.** Testes

_____ **4.** Thymus

_____ **5.** Parathyroid gland

_____ **6.** Hypothalamus

_____ **7.** Pancreas

_____ **8.** Ovaries

_____ **9.** Thyroid gland

_____ **10.** Pineal gland

a. produces melatonin

b. produces estrogen and progesterone

c. produces calcitonin and thyroxine

d. produces epinephrine and corticosteroids

e. produces insulin and glucagon

f. produces parathyroid hormone

g. produces several tropic hormone

h. produces several releasing and inhibiting hormones

i. produces thymosin

j. produces testosterone

Matching

_____ **1.** Testosterone

_____ **2.** Calcitonin

_____ **3.** Epinephrine

_____ **4.** Parathyroid hormone

_____ **5.** Insulin

_____ **6.** Estrogen

_____ **7.** Thyroxine

_____ **8.** Melatonin

_____ **9.** Glucagon

_____ **10.** Oxytocin

_____ **11.** TSH

_____ **12.** Thymosin

_____ **13.** Aldosterone

a. acts on the liver to increase blood sugar levels

b. regulates sleep/wake cycles

c. responds to chronic stressors

d. inhibits urine production

e. responsible for the production of milk

f. enhances male libido

g. responsible for "fight-or-flight" response

h. stimulates the thyroid gland

i. released in response to hyperglycemia

j. causes secondary sex characteristics in the female

k. causes maturation of T lymphocytes

l. helps regulate sodium balance

m. responsible for uterine contractions and milk let-down

_____ **14.** Prolactin

_____ **15.** Glucocorticoids

_____ **16.** ADH

_____ **17.** Progesterone

n. regulates uterine (menstrual) cycle

o. released in response to hypercalcemia

p. the main metabolic hormone of the body

q. acts on osteoclasts, kidneys, and intestines to increase blood calcium levels

Labeling

Draw your own lines and then label the following features on the diagram.

a. Pancreas

b. Ovaries

c. Pituitary gland

d. Adrenal glands

e. Thyroid gland

f. Testes

g. Hypothalamus

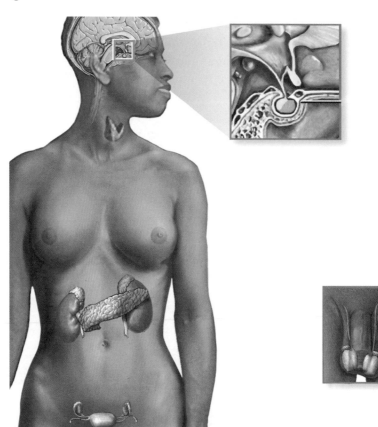

Fill in the Blank/Short Answer

1. As the "stress gland" the adrenal _____ responds to acute stress, whereas the adrenal _____ responds to chronic stress.

2. Hormones that act on other glands, causing them to secrete their own hormones are known as _____ hormones.

3. _____ glands secrete their products via a duct.

4. The "3 P's" of diabetes mellitus are the _____, _____, and

   _____.

5. The gland often referred to as the "master gland" is the _____.

6. The hypothalamus connects to the pituitary gland by a thin stalk known as the

   _____.

7. A diet deficient in _____ would interfere with the production of thyroid hormone

   causing an accumulation of colloid known as a _____.

8. The ability of the body to fight cancer is enhanced by hormones secreted from the

   _____ gland.

9. The hormone _____, released during childbirth, demonstrates a rare example of a

   positive feedback mechanism in the body.

10. Alcohol and caffeine interfere with the ability of ADH to autoregulate blood volume and osmolarity,

    often resulting in a case of excessive urination known as _____.

11. Juvenile or type _____ diabetes mellitus is considered an autoimmune condition.

Essay

1. Describe the three ways in which PTH helps to increase blood calcium levels in the body.

2. Describe the difference between diabetes insipidus and diabetes mellitus, including the glands and hormones involved in each.

3. Differentiate between the three forms of diabetes mellitus, including possible causes and treatments.

Cardiovascular System

6

Upon completion of this chapter, the student should be able to:

- Locate and describe the external anatomy of the heart and its great vessels
- Locate and describe the organization of the coronary blood vessels
- Locate and describe the internal anatomy of the heart including the chambers and valves
- Describe the pattern of systemic and pulmonary blood flow through the heart
- Locate the major blood vessels of the head and neck
- Identify the vessels that contribute to the Circle of Willis (cerebral arterial circle)
- Locate the major blood vessels of the upper extremity
- Locate the major blood vessels of the abdomen and describe hepatic portal circulation
- Locate the major vessels of the lower extremity

CARDIOVASCULAR SYSTEM OVERVIEW

The cardiovascular system is the main transportation system of the body. The heart is a thick, muscular organ equipped with a series of one-way valves to pump blood throughout the entire body. Dissolved in the blood are respiratory gases (oxygen and carbon dioxide), nutrients (glucose, amino acids, fatty acids, vitamins, etc.), wastes (lactic acid, urea), plasma proteins (antibodies, clotting factors, etc.), electrolytes (sodium, potassium, calcium, etc.), and hormones. This blood gets pumped through a series of blood vessels in order to deliver nutrients to the tissues and pick up wastes to be excreted. Arteries take blood away from the heart while veins transport blood back toward the heart. While most arteries are oxygenated and most veins are deoxygenated, the blood vessels are named for the direction of blood flow (either away from the heart or toward the heart), not the condition of the blood within their walls (oxygenated or deoxygenated). In this chapter, we review heart anatomy and take a look at the many blood vessels that serve the head and neck, torso, and upper and lower extremities.

LAB ACTIVITY 6.1

External Heart Anatomy

The heart is a muscular organ roughly the size of a closed fist located within the mediastinum, sandwiched between the lungs in the center of the thorax. The base of the heart is its superior border where most of the great vessels may be found entering and exiting the heart. The apex is pointed inferiorly and slightly off center to the left, lying just above the diaphragm. The heart is composed of three layers: the outer **epicardium** (or visceral pericardium), the middle **myocardium** (responsible for contraction), and the inner **endocardium** (a continuation of the vessel endothelial lining), which is in contact with the blood.

The heart contains four distinct chambers, which may be seen externally. The two superior chambers are known as **atria** (singular atrium) and are the receiving chambers. Oxygen-rich blood returning from the lungs enters the left atrium via four **pulmonary veins**. Deoxygenated blood returning from the rest of the body enters the right atrium via the **superior and inferior vena cavae**. The two inferior chambers are known as **ventricles** and act as the ejecting chambers. The right ventricle ejects deoxygenated blood to the lungs via the **pulmonary trunk** and **pulmonary arteries**. The left ventricle ejects oxygenated blood to systemic circulation via the **aorta**, the largest artery in the body. A small connective tissue remnant of fetal circulation known as the **ligamentum arteriosum** may be seen connecting the aorta to the pulmonary trunk. In fetal circulation, this patent connection was known as the **ductus arteriosus** and allowed for the shunting of blood between the two vessels. At birth, pressure changes in the thorax reroute blood flow causing this connection to close and become nonfunctional. Smaller blood vessels may also be found surrounding the external surface of the heart. These are the vessels of coronary circulation, which are discussed later.

Identify and label the base and apex of the heart as well as the great vessels associated with each heart chamber in the following figures.

To locate the image (anterior view) in AIA:
1. *Click on **Atlas Anatomy**; Select "**Thorax**," "**Cardiovascular**," "**Anterior**," and "**Illustration**" from the associated drop down menus.*
2. *Click "**Search**."*
3. *Find the image titled **Heart & Great Vessels (Ant).***

To locate the image (posterior view) in AIA:
1. *Click on **Atlas Anatomy**; Select "**Thorax**," "**Cardiovascular**," "**Posterior**," and "**Illustration**" from the associated drop down menus.*
2. *Click "**Search**."*
3. *Find the image titled **Heart & Great Vessels (Post).***

AA | Heart & Great Vessels (Ant)   AA | Heart & Great Vessels (Post)

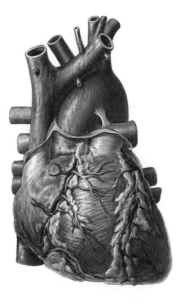
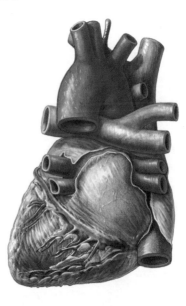

LAB ACTIVITY 6.2

Internal Heart Anatomy

Internally, the hollow chambers, septi, and valves may be visualized. The two atria are separated from each other by the thin **interatrial septum**. During fetal circulation, the lungs are filled with fluid so blood flows differently than it does after birth. Oxygenated blood comes to the heart via the umbilical cord in-utero rather than from the lungs. A hole in the interatrial septum, the **foramen ovale**, allows blood to flow between the atria during fetal circulation. Pressure changes within the thorax after birth allow for closure of this opening leaving a shallow depression in the interatrial septum known as the **fossa ovalis**. The two ventricles are separated by the thicker, more muscular **interventricular septum**. The thickness of the myocardium is more easily noticed in the internal view. Note the increased thickness of the left ventricular myocardium when compared to the right. The right ventricle only has to pump blood to the nearby lungs but the left ventricle must pump with more than five times the pressure of the right, ensuring adequate perfusion of the entire systemic circulation.

The heart contains four one-way valves, which ensure that blood flow stays unidirectional. The **atrioventricular (AV)** valves, as the name suggests, separate the superior atria from the inferior ventricles. The *right AV valve* has three cusps and is referred to as the **tricuspid valve**. It allows blood to flow from the right atrium into the right ventricle. The *left AV valve* has two cusps and is referred to as the **bicuspid** or **mitral** valve. It allows blood to flow from the left atrium into the left ventricle. With ventricular contraction, the AV valves are forced shut as pressure increases within the ventricles. This snapping shut of the AV valves may be heard (auscultated) as the "lub" sound or first sound of the heartbeat. Because these valves are under high pressure from the strongly contracting ventricles they are supported by small **papillary muscles** attached to thin, white cords known as **chordae tendineae**. These strong cords prevent the cusps of the AV valves from inverting back into the atria and ensure that blood exits the ventricles into either the pulmonary trunk or aorta. Because the left ventricle contracts with so much more force than the right, it is often the mitral valve that is damaged as a result of chronic cardiovascular diseases such as hypertension. The other set of valves are known as **semilunar valves** and may be found separating the ventricles from the great vessels. The **pulmonary semilunar valve** separates the pulmonary trunk from the right ventricle while the **aortic semilunar valve** is found between the aorta and the left ventricle. These valves are under lower pressure than the AV valves so they do not require the chordae tendineae reinforcements. With ventricular contraction these valves are at rest to allow blood to exit the ventricles. As blood is forced into the aorta and pulmonary trunk the vessels stretch to accommodate the volume of blood. As the vessels then recoil to their resting state some blood pushes back against the semilunar valves, forcing them shut and allowing for the second heart sound ("dub"). While the heart is made of four independent chambers, the entire heart functions together as a whole to assure blood is continually moved forward through its closed circuit.

To observe an animated overview of the cardiac cycle, including the heartbeat, valves, and blood flow:
1. *Click on* **Clinical Animations***; Select* "**Thorax**," "**Cardiovascular**," *and* "**Cardiology**" *from the associated drop down menus.*
2. *Click* "**Search**."
3. *Find the animation titled* **Heartbeat.**

 Heartbeat

Identify and label the internal structures of the heart including the chambers, valves, papillary muscles, and chordae tendineae in the following figure.
To locate the image in AIA:
1. *Click on* **Clinical Illustrations***; Select* "**Thorax**," "**Cardiovascular**," "**Anterior**," "**Illustration**," *and* "Cardiology" *from the associated drop down menus.*
2. *Click* "**Search**."
3. *Find the image titled* **Heart Valves - Anterior.**

CI | Heart Valves—Anterior

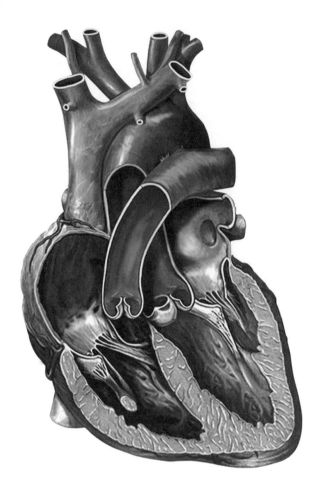

The following image allows you to visualize the thickness of the left ventricular myocardium.
To locate the image in AIA:
1. *Click on **Atlas Anatomy**; Select "**Thorax**," "**Cardiovascular**," "**Lateral**," and "**Illustration**" from the*
   associated drop down menus.
2. *Click "**Search**."*
3. *Find the image titled **Left Atrium & Ventricle (Lat)**.*

AA | Left Atrium & Ventricle (Lat)

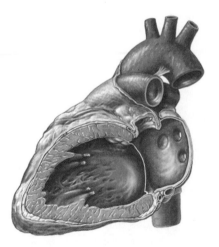

Compare as many structures as you can using the following images of the right side of the heart. To locate the images in AIA:

1. *Click on **Atlas Anatomy**; Select "**Thorax**," "**Cardiovascular**," "**Lateral**," and "**Illustration**" from the associated drop down menus.*
2. *Click "**Search**."*
3. *Find the image titled **Right Atrium (Lat).***

1. *Click on **Atlas Anatomy**; Select "**Thorax**," "**Cardiovascular**," "**Anterior**," and "**Cadaver Photograph**" from the associated drop down menus.*
2. *Click "**Search**."*
3. *Find the image titled **Right Atrium & Ventricle (Ant).***

AA Right Atrium (Lat)   **AA** Right Atrium & Ventricle (Ant)

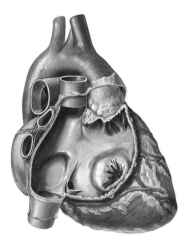
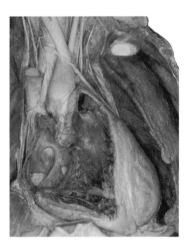

*For a unique interactive experience, click on the 3D Anatomy icon and then select **3D Heart**.*

3D Heart

From there you are able to manipulate a three-dimensional heart by rotating it, moving it, and zooming it in and out.

CLINICAL APPLICATIONS

There are several types of pathologies common to the heart. Conditions such as mitral or aortic stenosis involve a narrowing of the corresponding valve. This narrowing causes an increased resistance to blood flow thereby forcing the heart to contract with an increased pressure to overcome this resistance. The extra demand on the heart can lead to further complications such as cardiomyopathy or even heart failure.

To view some images of aortic and mitral stenosis in AIA:
1. *Click on Clinical Illustrations; Select "**Thorax**," "**Cardiovascular**," "**All**," "**Illustration**," and "**Cardiology**" from the associated drop down menus.*
2. *Click "**Search**."*
3. *Find the corresponding images.*

When heart valves become incompetent, that is they cannot close adequately or they invert in the opposite direction we find such conditions as mitral valve prolapse (MVP), aortic insufficiency, and tricuspid regurgitation. These conditions allow for the back-flow of blood and reduce the amount of blood moving through the heart correctly. In severe cases, it may be necessary to surgically repair or even replace the incompetent valve.

To view some images of valvular insufficiencies and heart valve replacements in AIA:
1. *Click on Clinical Illustrations; Select "**Thorax**," "**Cardiovascular**," "**All**," "**Illustration**," and "**Cardiology**" from the associated drop down menus.*
2. *Click "**Search**."*
3. *Find the corresponding images.*

Atrial and ventricular septal defects occur when there is an undesired opening in the septum connecting the right and left sides of the heart, allowing for the mixing of oxygenated and deoxygenated blood. When the foramen ovale fails to close properly, it is commonly referred to as a patent foramen ovale (PFO).

To view some images of atrial and ventricular septal defects in AIA:
1. *Click on* Clinical Illustrations*; Select* "***Thorax***," "***Cardiovascular***," "***All***," "***Illustration***," *and* "***Cardiology***" *from the associated drop down menus.*
2. *Click* "***Search***."
3. *Find the corresponding images.*

 LAB ACTIVITY 6.3

Circulation of Blood Through the Heart

The cardiovascular system is considered a "closed system," that is, blood is entirely contained within the walls of the heart and blood vessels (*plasma, white blood cells, and small nutrients/wastes may enter and leave circulation*). Since blood does not leave this system (*for our discussion purposes*), we can trace a drop of blood through the entire circulatory system and return it to the place where we began. Let's consider the two types of circulation in this closed system. "**Pulmonary circulation**" describes the flow of blood from the right side of the heart to the lungs and back to the left side of the heart, whereas "**Systemic circulation**" describes the flow of blood from the left side of the heart to the rest of the body systems and back to the right side of the heart. Let's begin our journey in the right atrium. From the right atrium we pass through the tricuspid valve into the right ventricle. Next, pass through the pulmonary semilunar valve into the pulmonary trunk, which then divides into the left and right pulmonary artery en route to the lungs. From the lungs, we enter the four pulmonary veins (two left and two right) and return to the left atrium. Next, pass through the bicuspid (mitral) valve into the left ventricle. From the left ventricle, pass through the aortic semilunar valve into the aorta, from which various systemic branches emerge to supply the body systems. Blood returning from the head, neck, and upper extremities enters the superior vena cava while blood returning from the thorax, abdomen, and lower extremities enters the inferior vena cava. Both the SVC and IVC enter into the right atrium of the heart, which is where we began in this example.

Use the following figure to trace blood flow through systemic and pulmonary circulation.
To locate the image in AIA:
1. *Click on* **Clinical Illustrations**; *Select* "***Thorax***," "***Cardiovascular***," "***Anterior***," "***Illustration***," *and* "*Cardiology*" *from the associated drop down menus.*
2. *Click* "***Search***."
3. *Find the image titled* **Circulation of Blood through the Heart.**

CI | Circulation of Blood Through the Heart

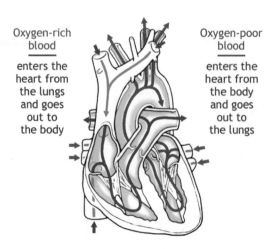

Oxygen-rich blood
———
enters the heart from the lungs and goes out to the body

Oxygen-poor blood
———
enters the heart from the body and goes out to the lungs

CLINICAL APPLICATIONS

While cardiac physiology is not discussed in detail here, the electrical activity of the heart is commonly analyzed in clinical practice. Electrocardiography is the act of recording the electrical activity of the heart to monitor cardiac function and check for pathology. An electrocardiogram (ECG) may be easily recorded in the hospital setting, in an ambulance, and even in most any physician's office.

1. Click on *Clinical Animations*; Select *"**Thorax**," "**Cardiovascular**," and "**Cardiology**"* from the associated drop down menus.
2. Click *"**Search**."*
3. Find the animations titled *"**Cardiac conduction system**" and "**Electrocardiogram (ECG)-interactive tool**."*

To view several images of ECG tracings in AIA:
1. Click on *Clinical Illustrations*; Select *"**Thorax**," "**Cardiovascular**," "**Non-standard**," "**Illustration**," and "**Cardiology**"* from the associated drop down menus.
2. Click *"**Search**."*
3. Find the corresponding images.

 LAB ACTIVITY 6.4

Coronary Blood Vessels

While the heart itself is filled with blood, the blood within the chambers does not supply the myocardium. Instead, the myocardium is supplied by a series of vessels that encircle the heart like a "crown," hence the name "**coronary**" vessels. The left and right coronary arteries are the two branches of the ascending aorta. When the ventricles contract these coronary arteries are actually compressed shut. Ventricular relaxation and the subsequent recoil of the aorta pushes blood back, closing the aortic valve, and forcing blood into the coronary arteries. Each coronary artery has two main, terminal branches. The **right coronary** artery gives rise to the **marginal artery** along the right lateral border of the heart, and then wraps around to the posterior aspect of the heart in the coronary sulcus (AV groove) and terminates in the **posterior interventricular artery**. The **left coronary** artery gives rise to the **anterior interventricular artery** and the **circumflex artery**. The circumflex artery wraps around the left side of the heart in the coronary sulcus. The anterior interventricular artery, also known as the **left anterior descending (LAD) artery** supplies the majority of the left ventricular myocardium. This vessel is referred to as the "widowmaker" by many cardiologists because a blood clot in this vessel often leads to left ventricular failure (infarct) followed by death. Drainage of myocardial blood is via cardiac, not coronary, veins. The **small cardiac vein** parallels the marginal artery and the **great cardiac vein** follows the reverse course of the anterior interventricular and circumflex arteries. The **middle cardiac vein** is found on the posterior aspect of the heart beside the posterior interventricular artery. The small, great, and middle cardiac veins drain into a common expanded vessel known as the **coronary sinus**, which then empties directly into the right atrium. Several anterior cardiac veins also empty directly into the right atrium from the anterior aspect of the heart.

Identify and label the coronary arteries and their branches in the following figures.
To locate the image (anterior view) in AIA:
1. Click on **Atlas Anatomy**; Select *"**Thorax**," "**Cardiovascular**," "**Anterior**," and "**Illustration**"* from the associated drop down menus.
2. Click *"**Search**."*
3. Find the image titled **Coronary Arteries (Ant).**

To locate the image (posterior view) in AIA:
1. Click on **Atlas Anatomy**; Select *"**Thorax**," "**Cardiovascular**," "**Posterior**," and "**Illustration**"* from the associated drop down menus.
2. Click *"**Search**."*
3. Find the image titled **Coronary Arteries (Post).**

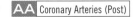

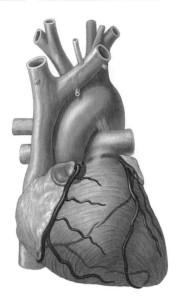
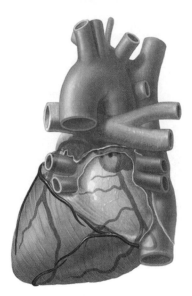

Identify and label the cardiac veins and the coronary sinus in the following figures.

To locate the image (anterior view) in AIA:

1. *Click on* **Atlas Anatomy**; *Select* **"Thorax,"** **"Cardiovascular,"** **"Anterior,"** *and* **"Illustration"** *from the associated drop down menus.*
2. *Click* **"Search."**
3. *Find the image titled* **Cardiac Veins (Ant).**

To locate the image (posterior view) in AIA:

1. *Click on* **Atlas Anatomy**; *Select* **"Thorax,"** **"Cardiovascular,"** **"Posterior,"** *and* **"Illustration"** *from the associated drop down menus.*
2. *Click* **"Search."**
3. *Find the image titled* **Cardiac Veins (Post).**

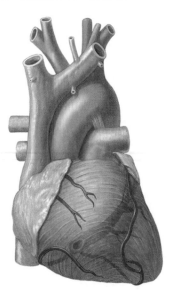
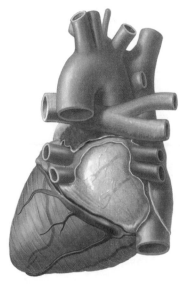

To examine images of the coronary arteries and cardiac veins from the superior view you may go to
Coronary Arteries (Sup) and Cardiac Veins (Sup)

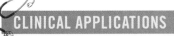

CLINICAL APPLICATIONS

Cardiac tissue, being aerobic, is very sensitive to oxygen and any interruption of blood flow (ischemia) has the potential to cause damage. Temporary ischemia frequently causes a sensation of pressure or squeezing chest pain known as angina pectoris. The symptoms are often eliminated with rest and there is no residual damage to the myocardial tissue. When muscle cells die from a lack of oxygen, a myocardial infarction (MI) or "heart attack" results. Heart attacks often occur as a result of severe coronary artery disease (CAD) although emboli lodging in the coronary vessels are another cause. While heart attacks do cause permanent damage, they are not always fatal. The amount and location of damaged tissue and the ability of the surrounding tissue to compensate for the lost (dead) tissue dictate the severity. Three common treatments for CAD are coronary artery bypass grafts (CABG), percutaneous transluminal coronary angioplasty (PTCA), and directional coronary atherectomy (DCA).

1. *Click on* Clinical Animations; *Select* "**Thorax**," "**Cardiovascular**," *and* "**Cardiology**" *from the associated drop down menus.*
2. *Click* "**Search**."
3. *Find the animations titled* "**Coronary artery bypass grafts (CABG)**," "**Percutaneous transluminal coronary angioplasty (PTCA)**," *and* "**Directional coronary atherectomy (DCA)**."

To view several images of CAD, MI, Angina, Angioplasty, and CABG in AIA:
1. *Click on* Clinical Illustrations; *Select* "**Thorax**," "**Cardiovascular**," "**All**," "**All**," *and* "**Cardiology**" *from the associated drop down menus.*
2. *Click* "**Search**."
3. *Find the corresponding images.*

 LAB ACTIVITY 6.5

Vessels of the Head and Neck

The aortic arch has three major branches that emerge to supply the head, neck, and upper extremities. The first branch of the aortic arch is the **brachiocephalic trunk**. Shortly after emerging from the aorta the brachiocephalic (brachio-"arm"/cephalic-"head") trunk divides to form the **right subclavian artery** serving the right upper extremity and the **right common carotid artery** serving the right side of the head and neck. The second branch emerging from the arch is the **left common carotid artery,** which serves the left side of the head and neck. The third and final branch of the aortic arch is the **left subclavian artery,** which supplies the left upper extremity. The subclavian arteries give off an additional branch that supplies the brain, the **vertebral artery**. The vertebral artery may be found ascending the neck through the transverse foramina of the cervical spine. The common carotid arteries (commonly used as pulse points) divide into the **internal carotid arteries,** which go on to serve the brain and the **external carotid arteries,** which serve the skin and muscles of the head and neck. Terminal branches of the external carotid arteries include the **occipital**, **superficial temporal**, and **facial arteries**.

Corresponding veins with the same names are found running with most arteries of the head and neck. A noticeable difference is with the carotids themselves since we have no named carotid veins. Instead, we have the **internal jugular vein** and **external jugular vein** that drain the respective areas supplied by the carotid arteries.

Identify and label the arteries of the head and neck in the following figure.
To locate the image in AIA:
1. *Click on* **Atlas Anatomy**; *Select* "**Head and Neck**," "**Cardiovascular**," "**Lateral**," *and* "**Illustration**" *from the associated drop down menus.*
2. *Click* "**Search**."
3. *Find the image titled* **Arteries of Head & Neck.**

AA Arteries of Head & Neck

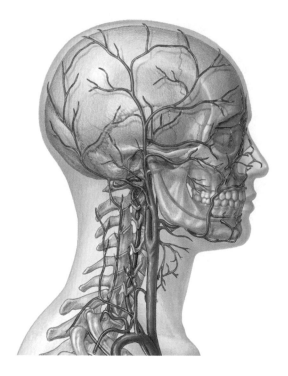

Identify and label the veins of the head and neck in the following figure.

To locate the image in AIA:

1. Click on **Atlas Anatomy**; Select "**Head and Neck**," "**Cardiovascular**," "**Lateral**," and "**Illustration**" from the associated drop down menus.

2. Click "**Search**."

3. Find the image titled **Veins of Head & Neck (Lat).**

AA Veins of Head & Neck (Lat)

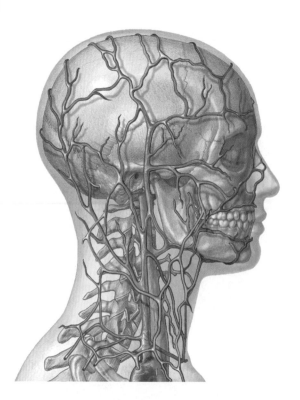

Since the neural tissue of the brain is perhaps the most oxygen-sensitive tissue in the body, there is a special blood supply to ensure that oxygen delivery to the brain is uninterrupted. The **cerebral arterial circle**, or *circle of Willis*, is an anastomosis of four major vessels: the left & right vertebral arteries entering the cranial vault via the foramen magnum and the left and right internal carotid arteries entering via the carotid canal of the temporal bone. These interconnected vessels are then arranged in a circle surrounding the pituitary gland, further dividing to supply the neural tissue of the brain. The internal carotid arteries branch to give us the **anterior** and **middle cerebral arteries**, while the vertebral arteries fuse to become the **basilar artery**. The basilar artery later divides to form the **posterior cerebral arteries**.

Identify and label the arteries of the cerebral arterial circle in the following figure.
To locate the image in AIA:
1. *Click on **Atlas Anatomy**; Select "**Head and Neck**," "**Cardiovascular**," "**Inferior**," and "**Illustration**" from the associated drop down menus.*
2. *Click "**Search**."*
3. *Find the image titled **Cerebral Arterial Circle (Inf)**.*

AA | Cerebral Arterial Circle (Inf)

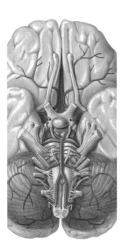

CLINICAL APPLICATIONS

When blood supply to a part of the brain is interrupted causing brain cells to die we call the condition a cerebrovascular accident (CVA), or stroke. Stroke patients often present with unilateral paralysis or loss of strength and difficulty with speech. A stroke is a medical emergency, and permanent disability or death can result if treatment is not initiated rapidly. A transient ischemic attack (TIA) is sometimes referred to as a "mini-stroke" but symptoms typically subside within 24 hours and do not result in permanent damage. TIAs are considered a serious warning sign of a stroke and should not be ignored.

1. *Click on Clinical Animations; Select "**Head and Neck**," "**Cardiovascular**," and "**Cardiology**" from the associated drop down menus.*
2. *Click "**Search**."*
3. *Find the animations titled **Stroke** and **Stroke - Secondary to Cardiogenic Embolism**.*

To view several images related to strokes in AIA:
1. *Click on Clinical Illustrations; Select "**Head and Neck**," "**Cardiovascular**," "**All**," "**All**," and "**All**" from the associated drop down menus.*
2. *Click "**Search**."*
3. *Find the corresponding images.*

In the following view of the deep veins of the head, specialized veins known as **dural venous sinuses** may be visualized. These sinuses are sandwiched between two layers of dura mater and collect venous blood from the brain as well as cerebrospinal fluid from the subarachnoid space as it gets reabsorbed into circulation. The dural venous sinuses eventually merge into the left and right internal jugular veins and exit the skull through the jugular foramen.

Identify and label the internal jugular vein and a few of the more prominent dural venous sinuses in the following figure.

To locate the image in AIA:

*1. Click on **Atlas Anatomy**; Select "**Head and Neck**," "**Cardiovascular**," "**Lateral**," and "**Illustration**" from the associated drop down menus.*

*2. Click "**Search**."*

*3. Find the image titled **Deep Veins of Head (Lat).***

AA | Deep Veins of Head (Lat)

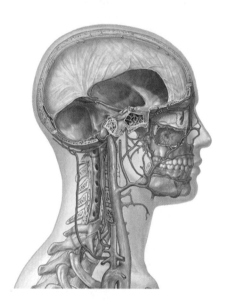

 LAB ACTIVITY 6.6

Vessels of the Upper Extremity

The arch of the aorta gives rise to the arteries that supply the upper extremity. The **right subclavian artery** divides from the **brachiocephalic trunk** whereas the **left subclavian artery** is the third and final branch of the aortic arch. The subclavian artery then continues on and becomes the **axillary artery,** which serves the axilla, shoulder, and part of the lateral chest wall. It continues as the **brachial artery,** which supplies the musculature of the arm before dividing at the elbow into the **radial** (commonly used as a pulse point) and **ulnar arteries,** which serve the forearm. These two vessels then enter the hand as the **superficial** and **deep palmar arches**.

The deep veins of the upper extremity run opposite to their arterial counterparts. The **superficial** and **deep palmar arches** continue into the forearm as the **radial** and **ulnar veins**. These then merge into the **brachial vein,** which then empties into the **axillary vein**. The axillary vein continues as the **subclavian vein** which, after uniting with the **internal jugular vein**, becomes the **brachiocephalic vein**. The left and right brachiocephalic veins then merge into the **superior vena cava,** which enters the heart at the right atrium.

Identify and label the vessels of the upper extremity in the following figures.

To locate the image in AIA:

*1. Click on **Atlas Anatomy**; Select "**Upper Limb**," "**Cardiovascular**," "**Anterior**," and "**Illustration**" from the associated drop down menus.*

*2. Click "**Search**."*

*3. Find the image titled **Arteries of Upper Limb (Ant).***

To locate the image in AIA:

1. *Click on* **Atlas Anatomy**; *Select* "**Upper Limb**," "**Cardiovascular**," "**Anterior**," *and* "**Illustration**" *from the associated drop down menus.*
2. *Click "***Search***."*
3. *Find the image titled* **Deep Veins of Upper Limb (Ant).**

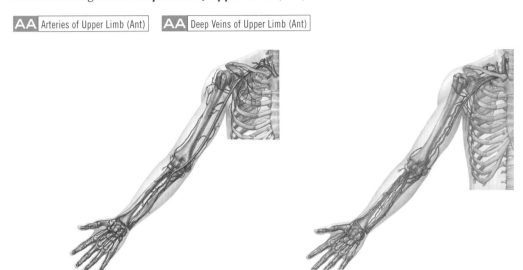

Superficially, the upper extremity has a network of veins with no arterial partners. The **cephalic vein** may be found running along the lateral forearm and arm before joining into the axillary vein in the area of the shoulder. The **basilic vein** runs along the medial forearm and arm before entering the deeper, brachial vein. The basilic and cephalic veins unite at the antecubital fossa (anterior elbow) to form the **median cubital vein,** which is a common site used for blood removal (phlebotomy) and IV administration.

Identify and label the superficial veins of the upper extremity in the following figure. Zooming in will allow you to view the extremity in its entirety. To view the image in AIA, go to

 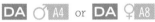 or

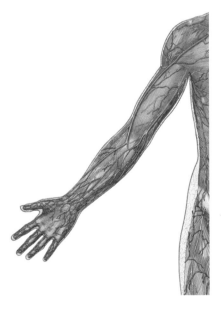

LAB ACTIVITY 6.7

Branches of the Descending Aorta

As the aorta turns downward from the arch it becomes the ***descending aorta***. The section of descending aorta superior to the diaphragm is known as the ***thoracic aorta***. The branches of the thoracic aorta include intercostal arteries plus branches to the esophagus, lungs, and diaphragm. As the descending aorta passes through the diaphragm its name changes from the thoracic aorta to the ***abdominal aorta***.

The first main branch of the abdominal aorta is the **celiac trunk**. Almost immediately the celiac trunk divides into three vessels: the **common hepatic artery** to the liver, the **left gastric artery** to the stomach, and the **splenic artery** to the spleen.

The **superior mesenteric artery** is a singular vessel supplying the majority of the small intestine and the proximal portion of the large intestine (colon).

The paired **renal arteries** supply the left and right kidneys and give off smaller **suprarenal** branches to the adrenal glands sitting atop of each kidney.

The next branches are the paired ***gonadal arteries*** serving either the testes or ovaries. In a male, these are known as the **testicular arteries** while in the female, they are called the **ovarian arteries**.

Finally, the singular **inferior mesenteric artery** may be found supplying the distal half of the large intestine.

Identify and label the branches of the abdominal aorta in the following figure. To locate the image in AIA:
1. *Click on **Atlas Anatomy**; Select "**Body Wall and Back**," "**Cardiovascular**," "**Anterior**," and "**Illustration**" from the associated drop down menus.*
2. *Click "**Search**."*
3. *Find the image titled **Arteries of Trunk (Ant)**.*

AA Arteries of Trunk (Ant)

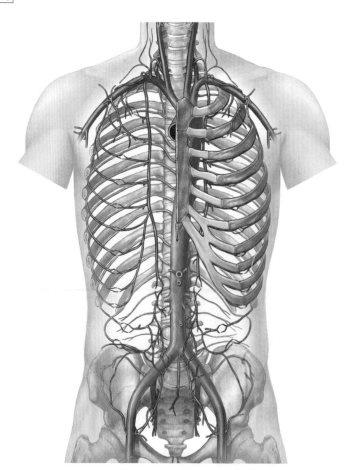

The following images show close-up views of the branches of the celiac trunk as well as the superior mesenteric artery.

Compare as many structures as you can using the following images of the abdominal viscera. To locate the image in AIA:
1. *Click on* **Atlas Anatomy**; *Select "**Abdomen**," "**Cardiovascular**," "**Anterior**," and "**Illustration**" from the associated drop down menus.*
2. *Click "**Search**."*
3. *Find the image titled* **Superior Mesenteric Artery 1.**

To locate the image in AIA:
1. *Click on* **Atlas Anatomy**; *Select "**Abdomen**," "**Cardiovascular**," "**Anterior**," and "**Cadaver Photograph**" from the associated drop down menus.*
2. *Click "**Search**."*
3. *Find the image titled* **Pancreas & Spleen (Ant).**

AA Superior Mesenteric Artery 1   AA Pancreas & Spleen (Ant)

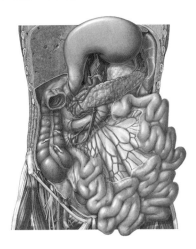 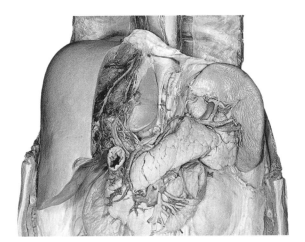

For a closer look at the distribution of the inferior mesenteric artery:
1. *Click on* **Atlas Anatomy**; *Select "**Abdomen**," "**Cardiovascular**," "**Anterior**," and "**Illustration**" from the associated drop down menus.*
2. *Click "**Search**."*
3. *Find the image titled* **Inferior Mesenteric Artery 1.**

AA Inferior Mesenteric Artery 1

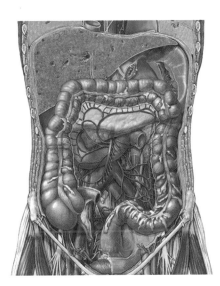

Veins of the Abdomen

The **inferior vena cava** receives blood from the organs of the abdomen as well as the lower extremities. The left and right **hepatic veins**, draining the liver, enter the inferior vena cava just inferior to the diaphragm. The **renal veins** may be seen prominently entering the inferior vena cava, draining the left and right kidneys. The **right suprarenal vein** connects directly to the inferior vena cava while the **left suprarenal vein** joins with the left renal vein. Similarly, the **right gonadal vein** enters the inferior vena cava directly whereas the **left gonadal vein** joins the left renal vein. The remaining organs have their blood collected by the hepatic portal circulation, which is discussed in the next section.

Identify and label the vessels draining into the inferior vena cava in the following figure. To view the image in AIA, go to

  or

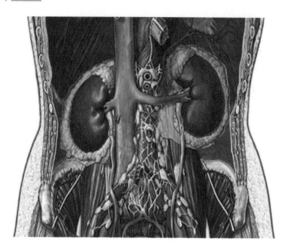

LAB ACTIVITY 6.9

Hepatic Portal Circulation

The liver is a multifunctional organ with hundreds of different functions. It is a production factory, a storage facility, and a waste removal plant all rolled into one. As such, it is important that the liver has access to ingested nutrients as well as potential ingested toxins. A special circulatory pathway known as ***hepatic portal circulation*** is responsible for collecting blood from the digestive organs, pancreas, and spleen, and then delivering the blood to the liver for processing. The **inferior mesenteric vein**, carrying blood from the colon, joins with the **splenic vein,** which contains blood from the spleen, pancreas, and stomach. The **superior mesenteric vein**, with its blood from the small intestine and proximal colon, unites with the splenic vein to form the **hepatic portal vein,** which then enters the liver from its inferior surface. The liver will store or process the carried nutrients, preparing them for delivery to general circulation. The **left** and **right hepatic veins** then exit the liver and join the **inferior vena cava**.

Identify and label the vessels of hepatic circulation in the following figure. To locate the image in AIA:
1. *Click on **Atlas Anatomy**; Select "**Abdomen**," "**Cardiovascular**," "**Anterior**," and "**Illustration**" from the associated drop down menus.*
2. *Click "**Search**."*
3. *Find the image titled **Mesenteric Veins**.*

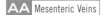

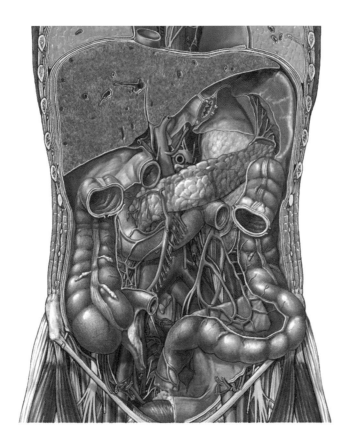

The following images show close-up views of the hepatic portal vein as well as the mesenteric and splenic veins.
Compare as many structures as you can using the following images of the abdominal viscera. To locate the image in AIA:
1. Click on **Atlas Anatomy**; Select "**Abdomen**," "**Cardiovascular**," "**Anterior**," and "**Illustration**" from the associated drop down menus.
2. Click "**Search**."
3. Find the image titled **Hepatic Portal Vein.**

To locate the image in AIA:
1. Click on **Atlas Anatomy**; Select "**Abdomen**," "**Cardiovascular**," "**Anterior**," and "**Cadaver Photograph**" from the associated drop down menus.
2. Click "**Search**."
3. Find the image titled **Dissection of Portal Vein.**

AA | Hepatic Portal Vein   AA | Dissection of Portal Vein

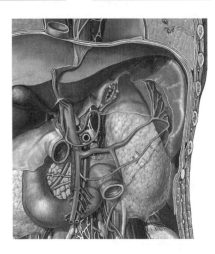 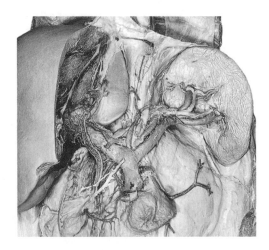

 LAB ACTIVITY 6.10

Vessels of the Lower Extremity

Once the abdominal aorta reaches the level of approximately L4 it terminates and divides into the **left** and **right common iliac arteries**. The common iliac arteries soon divide into the **internal iliac artery,** which supplies the organs of the pelvis (bladder, rectum, prostate in males, and vagina in females), gluteal muscles, and the adductor muscles of the thigh. The **external iliac artery** supplies blood to the skin and muscles of the lower abdomen before exiting the pelvis to supply the lower limb. In the thigh, its name changes to the **femoral artery** where it supplies the femur and muscles of the thigh. Branching from the proximal portion of the femoral artery is the **deep femoral artery,** which supplies the majority of the thigh musculature. Branching from this vessel are the **lateral** and **medial circumflex femoral arteries**, supplying the areas around the head and neck of the femur. At the knee, the femoral artery continues on as the **popliteal artery,** which then divides into the **anterior** and **posterior tibial arteries,** which supply the leg. The anterior tibial artery crosses the ankle joint as the **dorsalis pedis artery** (terminating as the **dorsal arcuate artery**) while the posterior tibial artery wraps around the posterior aspect of the medial malleolus, terminating as the **medial** and **lateral plantar arteries**. Both the dorsalis pedis and posterior tibial arteries are common pulse points in the lower extremity.

Blood from the plantar aspect of the foot enters the **posterior tibial vein** while that of the dorsum of the foot enters the **anterior tibial vein**. The anterior and posterior tibial veins join to form the **popliteal vein** at the knee, which then continues up the thigh as the **femoral vein**. Once in the pelvis, the femoral vein becomes the **external iliac vein,** which will then join with the **internal iliac vein** to become the **common iliac vein**. The left and right common iliac veins unite to form the **inferior vena cava,** which ascends the abdomen to enter the heart via the right atrium.

Identify and label the vessels of the thigh in the following figures. To locate the image in AIA:

1. *Click on **Atlas Anatomy**; Select "**Lower Limb**," "**Cardiovascular**," "**Anterior**," and "**Illustration**" from the associated drop down menus.*
2. *Click "**Search**."*
3. *Find the image titled **Arteries of Lower Limb (Ant)**.*

To locate the image in AIA:

1. *Click on **Atlas Anatomy**; Select "**Lower Limb**," "**Cardiovascular**," "**Anterior**," and "**Illustration**" from the associated drop down menus.*
2. *Click "**Search**."*
3. *Find the image titled **Deep Veins of Lower Limb (Ant).***

AA Arteries of Lower Limb (Ant)   **AA** Deep Veins of Lower Limb (Ant)

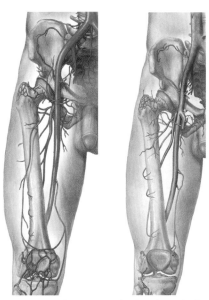

Using the same two previous illustrations, scroll down to the level of the leg and identify the vessels of the leg and foot.

AA Arteries of Lower Limb (Ant)   **AA** Deep Veins of Lower Limb (Ant)

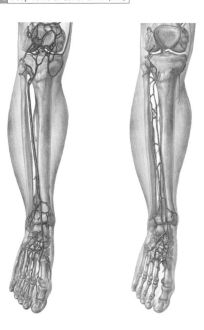

For a better view of the posterior leg vasculature, use the following figures to identify and label the vessels of the posterior leg. To locate the image in AIA:
1. *Click on **Atlas Anatomy**; Select "**Lower Limb**," "**Cardiovascular**," "**Posterior**," and "**Illustration**" from the associated drop down menus.*
2. *Click "**Search**."*
3. *Find the image titled **Arteries of Lower Limb (Post).***

To locate the image in AIA:
1. *Click on **Atlas Anatomy**; Select "**Lower Limb**," "**Cardiovascular**," "**Posterior**," and "**Illustration**" from the associated drop down menus.*
2. *Click "**Search**."*
3. *Find the image titled **Deep Veins of Lower Limb (Post).***

AA Arteries of Lower Limb (Post)   **AA** Deep Veins of Lower Limb (Post)

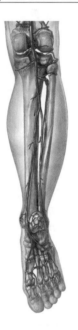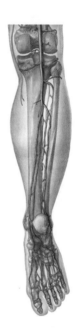

Superficially, the lower extremity has a network of veins with no arterial partners. The **small saphenous vein** may be found coursing from lateral aspect of the foot and up the posterior leg before joining with the **popliteal vein** behind the knee. The **great saphenous vein** is the longest vein in the human body and takes a long, tortuous route along the entire lower extremity. It originates from the medial side of the dorsum of the foot, and then progresses along the medial leg and thigh before joining the deeper, **femoral vein** just below the inguinal ligament. The great saphenous vein is a common site for harvesting grafts to be used for CABG procedures.

To view the superficial veins of the lower extremity in AIA go to
DA ♂ P3 *or* **DA** ♀ P3 *to visualize the small saphenous vein and go to* **DA** ♂ A5 *or* **DA** ♀ A8 *to get a good view of the great saphenous vein. Zooming in and out and scrolling up and down will allow you to view the extremity and its vessels in their entirety.*

CARDIOVASCULAR SYSTEM REVIEW EXERCISES

Matching

_____ **1.** Right AV valve

_____ **2.** CVA

_____ **3.** Vessel used when taking blood pressure

_____ **4.** Commonly used in CABG procedures

_____ **5.** Angina pectoris

_____ **6.** Common site for pulse

_____ **7.** LAD

_____ **8.** Left AV valve

a. radial artery

b. mitral valve

c. anterior interventricular artery

d. chest pain

e. brachial artery

f. great saphenous vein

g. tricuspid valve

h. stroke

Labeling

Draw your own lines and then label following features on the diagram.

a. Right coronary artery

b. Left pulmonary artery

c. Left common carotid artery

d. Brachiocephalic trunk

e. Inferior vena cava

f. Left brachiocephalic vein

g. Anterior interventricular artery

h. Superior vena cava

i. Pulmonary trunk

j. Left subclavian vein

k. Ligamentum arteriosum

l. Right pulmonary veins

m. Aortic arch

n. Great cardiac vein

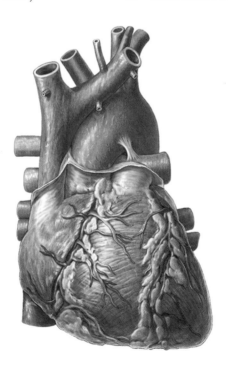

Draw your own lines and then label following features on the diagram.

a. Left common carotid artery
b. Right common iliac artery
c. Celiac trunk
d. Brachiocephalic trunk
e. Right renal artery
f. Inferior mesenteric artery
g. Right vertebral artery

h. Left axillary artery
i. Left internal iliac artery
j. Thoracic aorta
k. Superior mesenteric artery
l. Left gonadal artery
m. Right external iliac artery

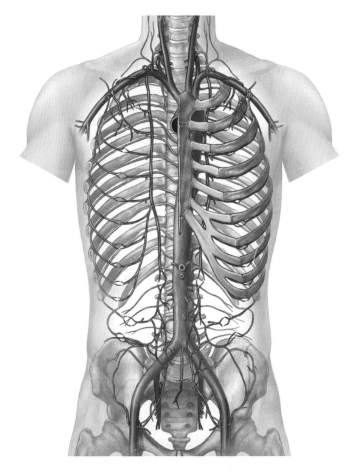

Draw your own lines and then label following features on the diagram.

a. Inferior mesenteric vein   **e.** Superior mesenteric vein

b. Right external iliac vein   **f.** Left common iliac vein

c. Splenic vein   **g.** Hepatic portal vein

d. Inferior vena cava   **h.** Left femoral vein

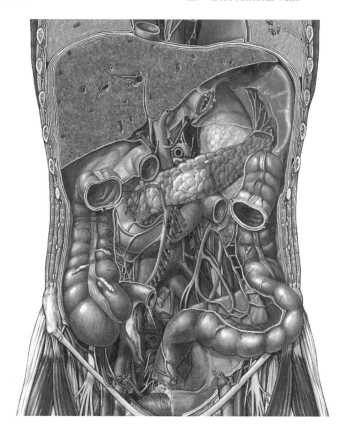

Fill in the Blank/Short Answer

1. The gonadal artery in the female is better known as the _____ artery.

2. The radial and ulnar vein merge to form the _____ vein.

3. The two major arteries supplying the brain are the _____ and _____.

4. The middle and great cardiac veins drain into the _____, which then enters the right atrium.

5. The longest vein in the body is the _____.

6. The inner lining of the heart in contact with the blood is the _____.

7. The second branch of the aortic arch is the _____.

8. The most common site for venipuncture is the _____ vein.

9. The pulse of the _____ artery may easily be palpated on the dorsum of the foot.

10. The _____ valve separates the left atrium from the left ventricle.

11. The opening in the interatrial septum normally found during fetal circulation is the

    _____.

12. The veins draining the digestive organs, pancreas, and spleen collectively enter the liver via the

    _____.

13. The interconnected network of vessels supplying the brain with oxygenated blood is known as the

    _____.

14. The role of the chordae tendineae is to _____.

15. Incomplete closure of the tricuspid valve would cause blood to back up into _____.

Essay

1. Beginning with the left ventricle, trace a drop of blood through the entire cardiovascular system, returning to the left ventricle. (Be sure to include valves, chambers, and great vessels).

2. Beginning with the large intestine, trace a drop of blood back to the right atrium. (Be sure to include vessels and organs encountered along the way).

3. Compare and contrast a TIA with a CVA.

Lymphatic System

7

LEARNING OBJECTIVES

Upon completion of this chapter, the student should be able to:

- Describe the two primary functions of the lymphatic system
- Locate and describe the major tissues and glands associated with the lymphatic system
- Describe the basic pattern of lymphatic drainage
- Locate and describe the cervical lymph nodes
- Locate and describe the function of the thymus gland
- Locate the cisterna chyli and describe its connection to the thoracic duct
- Identify the spleen and describe its role in the lymphatic system
- Locate and describe the inguinal lymph nodes

LYMPHATIC SYSTEM OVERVIEW

The lymphatic system has two distinct, very important functions to carry out in the body. The first is to reclaim fluids that have leaked out of the cardiovascular system and transport them back into systemic circulation. This is accomplished via a vast network of lymphatic vessels that are intimately associated with the cardiovascular system. The second vital function is to provide for our body's immune response. Various lymphatic tissues and organs containing specialized lymphocytes and phagocytic cells are scattered throughout the body to help keep us resistant to disease and protect us from infection and abnormal (cancer) cell growth.

CI Immune System Structures

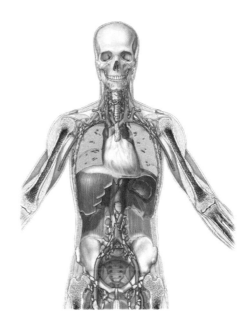

LAB ACTIVITY 7.1

Lymphatic Circulation

Unlike the cardiovascular system, which has a cyclical circulation pattern (heart → arteries → capillaries → veins → heart), lymphatic circulation flows in one direction only, from distal to proximal. There is no comparable pump to help propel the lymph so lymphatic vessels must rely on thoracic and abdominal pressure changes, skeletal muscle contraction, and specialized, one-way valves to keep lymph flowing unidirectionally toward the heart. With few exceptions, lymphatic capillaries are found almost everywhere systemic capillaries are located. Hydrostatic pressure from within the cardiovascular system forces nutrients and plasma across the capillary walls in order to nourish our body tissues. While much of the fluid is reclaimed by the capillaries, some remains in the tissues as interstitial fluid. If this interstitial fluid had no mechanism to return to general circulation, it wouldn't take long for the cardiovascular system to shut down from a lack of blood volume. As the interstitial fluid is reclaimed into lymphatic capillaries, it becomes lymph and begins its trek back to general circulation. **Lymphatic capillaries** merge into lymphatic vessels, which then proceed through a vast collection of lymph nodes that serve to filter the lymph and remove undesirable microorganisms before they have an opportunity to enter the bloodstream. The meandering network of **lymph vessels** then merge into fewer, larger collections of **lymphatic trunks** that are named for their locations in the body, that is, bronchomediastinal, intestinal, lumbar, etc. Ultimately, all of the named trunks enter into one of two lymphatic ducts—the **right lymphatic duct** or the **thoracic duct**. The right lymphatic duct drains lymph from the right side of the head, the right upper extremity, and the right side of the thorax. The thoracic duct originates at approximately the T12 vertebral level in an expansive sac known as the **cisterna chyli** and then progresses superiorly alongside of the vertebral column, collecting lymph from the entire rest of the body. Both of the ducts eventually enter into the subclavian vein on their respective sides of the body. Once the lymph enters into the subclavian vein, it has now re-entered systemic circulation and is once again known as plasma. The lymphatic system returns as much as 3 to 4 L of interstitial fluid to general circulation per day. Lymphatic obstruction may sometimes lead to a collection of interstitial fluid within the tissues known as **_edema_**.

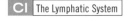 The Lymphatic System   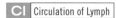 Circulation of Lymph

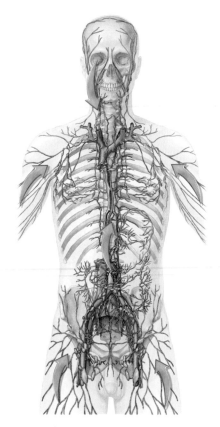

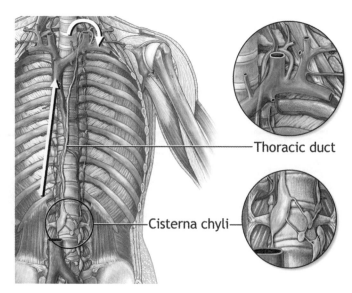

Thoracic duct

Cisterna chyli

Identify and label scattered lymph nodes, the cisterna chyli, and the thoracic duct in the following figure. To view the image in AIA, go to

 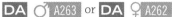 or

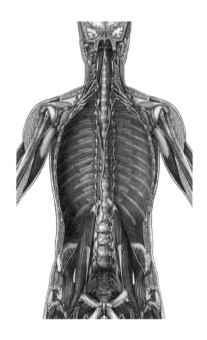

CLINICAL APPLICATIONS

Lymphocytes are white blood cells that have an important role in initiating and managing the immune response. ***T lymphocytes*** are responsible for cell-mediated (cell-to-cell interaction) immunity while ***B lymphocytes*** are responsible for humoral (antibody-mediated) immunity. In addition to lymphocytes, other types of white blood cells include neutrophils, monocytes, eosinophils, and basophils. While an in-depth discussion regarding the function of each of these cells is beyond the scope of this text, it is important to realize that each of these white blood cells has specific, but often overlapping, functions. Health care providers regularly order laboratory blood tests to look at the size, shape, color, and number of each type of blood cells in an effort to better diagnose disease.

To view some images of blood cells and white blood counts in AIA:
1. *Click on Clinical Illustrations; Select "**All**," "**Lymphatic**," "**All**," "**All**," and "**Allergy & Immunology**" from the associated drop down menus.*
2. *Click "**Search**."*
3. *Find the corresponding images.*

LAB ACTIVITY 7.2

The Lymph Nodes

As lymph flows through the lymphatic vessels toward its ultimate destination into systemic circulation, it gets filtered along the way by clusters of lymphoid tissue known as **lymph nodes**. Lymph nodes have more lymphatic vessels (**afferent vessels**) entering into them than they do (**efferent vessels**) exiting from them. This presentation slows lymphatic flow through the node allowing time for the lymph to be acted upon and filtered. It is the role of lymph nodes to filter the lymph of microorganisms such as bacteria and viruses, abnormal (cancer) cells, and other foreign debris before they have an opportunity to enter general circulation. While lymph nodes are scattered throughout the body, we find clusters of lymph nodes specifically located within the **cervical**, **axillary**, and **inguinal** regions. While we do not typically notice lymph nodes in a healthy state, as *lymphocytes* and *macrophages* housed within the nodes become more active with an infection, it is common to be able to palpate swollen lymph nodes in these superficial regions.

Identify and label the cervical lymph nodes and notice the lymphatic drainage patterns of the head and neck regions in the following figures. To locate the images in AIA:

1. *Click on* **Atlas Anatomy***; Select* "**Head and Neck**," "**Lymphatic**," "**All**," *and* "**Illustration**" *from the associated drop down menus.*
2. *Click* "**Search**."
3. *Find the images titled* **Lymph Flow of Head (Lat), Lymph Flow of Neck (Ant)**, *and* **Lymph Flow of Tongue (Dorsal)**.

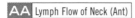

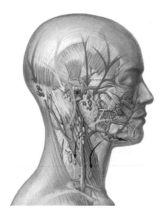

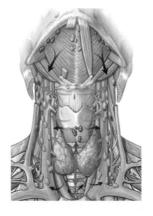

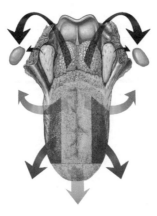

Identify and label some deeper bronchomediastinal and iliac lymph in the following figures. To locate the images in AIA:

1. *Click on **Atlas Anatomy**; Select "**Thorax**," "**Lymphatic**," "**All**," and "**Illustration**" from the associated drop down menus.*
2. *Click "**Search**."*
3. *Find the image titled **Lymph Nodes of Thorax (Ant)**.*

1. *Select "**Lower Limb**," "**Lymphatic**," "**All**," and "**Illustration**" from the associated drop down menus.*
2. *Click "**Search**."*
3. *Find the image titled **Contents of Femoral Triangle**.*

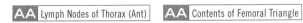

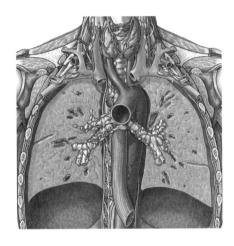
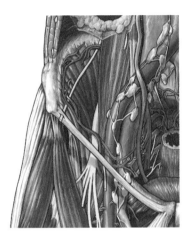

Identify and label the inguinal lymph nodes in the following figure. To view the image in AIA, go to

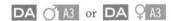

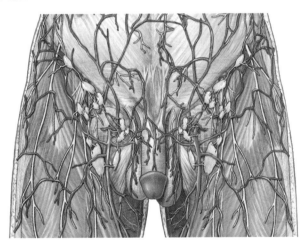

The Tonsils

The tonsils are collections of lymphatic tissue that are found within the pharyngeal mucosa. Tonsils are unencapsulated and serve to trap any microorganisms that may be unintentionally taken into the nose or mouth, thereby preventing them from entering into the respiratory tract. Located at the posterior aspect of the nasopharynx are the **pharyngeal tonsils**. Often, when the pharyngeal tonsils are inflamed, they are referred to as the *adenoids*. Located at the back of the oral cavity are found the **palatine tonsils**, wedged between the palatoglossal and palatopharyngeal arches (fauces). Finally, located at the base of the tongue are found the **lingual tonsils**.

Identify and label the pharyngeal and lingual tonsils in the following figure. To view the image in AIA, go to

  or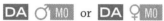

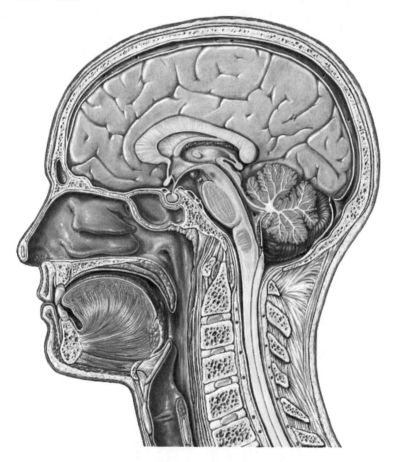

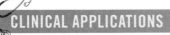

CLINICAL APPLICATIONS

An **allergy** is a condition in which a person responds to a substance (an *allergen*) that would not typically provoke an immune reaction in a healthy individual. Allergens may be contacted through the skin, inhaled into the lungs, swallowed, or even injected. Exposure to an allergen causes mast cells to release **histamine,** which is responsible for the majority of symptoms commonly associated with allergies. Allergy symptoms range from itchy eyes, runny noses, sneezing, and mild rashes. Some allergy sufferers choose to treat their symptoms by taking medication known as *antihistamine* to counter the effects of histamine. On occasion, allergies can cause much more serious and even life-threatening symptoms. **Anaphylaxis** is the term used to describe a life-threatening allergic reaction. Anaphylaxis causes a swelling of the throat and associated respiratory passages coupled with a drastic drop in blood pressure, eventually leading to a loss of consciousness. Those aware of their allergies often carry *epinephrine* to counter the effects of anaphylaxis. Epinephrine causes vasoconstriction (increases blood pressure) and bronchiole dilation (opens airways), which causes an almost immediate reversal of symptoms if administered properly and in the correct amount of time. Some medications (such as penicillin), bee stings, and even something as inconspicuous as a peanut have the ability to wreak havoc with the immune response. It is important to be able to recognize the signs of anaphylaxis in case you are ever called upon to help someone experiencing this life-threatening reaction.

To view some images of allergic reactions and anaphylaxis in AIA:
1. *Click on Clinical Illustrations; Select "**All**," "**Immune**," "**All**," "**All**," and "**Allergy & Immunology**" from the associated drop down menus.*
2. *Click "**Search**."*
3. *Find the corresponding images.*

 LAB ACTIVITY 7.4

The Thymus

The thymus is a lymphatic organ that can be found in the superior aspect of the mediastinum, just overlying the heart. While the thymus is rather large at birth, it is not very functional. The thymus reaches its peak function during childhood and then already begins to regress in function and atrophy around the time of adolescence. While maternal antibodies that have been passed through the placenta and then subsequently via breast feeding help protect the developing infant, once breast feeding ceases (typically after the first 12 months of life) thymus function increases as the infant begins to fight its own "immune system battles." The primary role of the thymus is to develop T lymphocytes, whose job is to distinguish between normal body cells and abnormal (virus infected, cancer) cells. The inability of the T lymphocytes to distinguish normal "self" from "nonself" may lead to a variety of autoimmune diseases and perhaps even the proliferation of cancer.

Identify and label the thymus in the following figure. To view the image in AIA, go to

  or

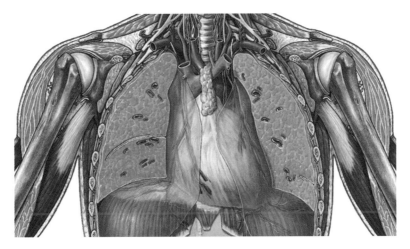

LAB ACTIVITY 7.5

The Spleen

While the lymphatic tissues discussed so far are responsible for filtering lymph, the spleen is the only lymphoid organ responsible for filtering blood. The spleen is located on the left side of the abdominal cavity, sitting directly below the diaphragm, and contains two distinct areas: **red pulp**, which is responsible for blood-cleansing functions and **white pulp**, which acts to mount immunological responses to antigens found within the blood and serves as a site for lymphocyte proliferation. Since all mucus membranes of the body opened to the outside contain mucosa-associated lymphatic tissue (MALT), the vast majority of microorganisms entering the body should be removed by the lymph before they ever reach the bloodstream, leaving little need for a major blood filter for microorganisms. The spleen also acts as a blood reservoir and with conditions that require additional blood volume the spleen can contract, emptying the blood reserve into general circulation. Sometimes, the contractions are even noticeable in what is commonly referred to as a "side stitch." Additionally, the spleen destroys aged red blood cells, stores platelets, and recycles iron for the liver to use in the manufacturing of new hemoglobin.

Identify and label the spleen in the following figure. To view the image in AIA, go to

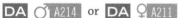 or

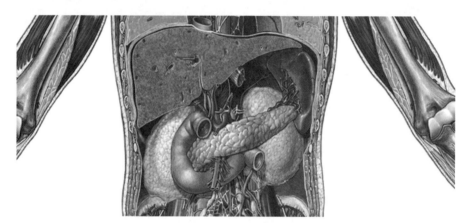

CLINICAL APPLICATIONS

Splenomegaly is a condition where the spleen becomes enlarged due to a host of different reasons. Infections, such as mononucleosis (the "kissing disease"), certain liver diseases, hemolytic anemia (the destruction of red blood cells), and even some cancers such as leukemia and Hodgkin disease may cause the spleen to enlarge. In most cases the effects on the spleen are only temporary. The spleen is also susceptible to trauma and is often damaged in cases of high-impact trauma such as with motor vehicle accidents (MVAs). Next time you sit in the driver's seat of an automobile, close the door and take notice to the level of the door handle in relation to your ribcage. It is easy to see how an impact from the side can traumatize this important blood-cleansing organ.

To view some images of splenomegaly and the effects of mononucleosis in AIA:
1. *Click on Clinical Illustrations; Select "All," "Lymphatic," "All," "All," and "Infectious Diseases" from the associated drop down menus.*
2. *Click "Search."*
3. *Find the corresponding images.*

LYMPHATIC SYSTEM REVIEW EXERCISES

Matching

_____ **1.** Thymus

_____ **2.** Right lymphatic duct

_____ **3.** Spleen

_____ **4.** Tonsils

_____ **5.** Thoracic duct

_____ **6.** Lymph nodes

_____ **7.** Cisterna chyli

_____ **8.** Lymphatic capillaries

a. drains lymph from the left side of head, left upper extremity, and below the abdomen

b. clusters of lymph tissue within the pharynx

c. the sac at the origin of the thoracic duct

d. responsible for developing T lymphocytes

e. associated with systemic capillaries and collect excess interstitial fluid

f. drains lymph from the right side of head and right upper extremity

g. filters lymph as it is transported toward the heart

h. filters blood and destroys worn out red blood cells

Labeling

Draw your own lines and then label the following features on the diagram.

a. Spleen

b. Inguinal lymph nodes

c. Thymus

d. Cervical lymph nodes

e. Axillary lymph nodes

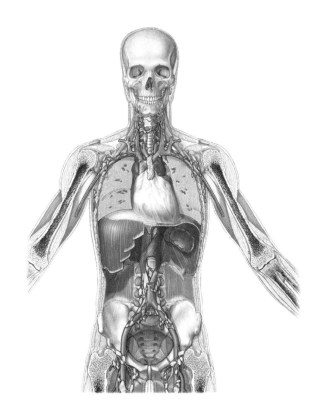

Fill in the Blank/Short Answer

1. A collection of interstitial fluid within the tissues is known as _____.

2. Two types of cells housed within lymph nodes are _____ and _____.

3. The spleen consists of _____ pulp that cleanses the blood and _____ pulp that mounts the immunological response to antigens in the bloodstream.

4. The lymphatic organ that reaches its peak during childhood and then begins to decline in function is the _____.

5. The _____ tonsils are found in the nasopharynx while the _____ tonsils are found in the oral cavity.

6. Lymph originating from the head and neck is likely to filter through the _____ lymph nodes while lymph from the foot will filter through the _____ nodes.

7. Lymphatic vessels contain one-way _____ to assist moving the lymph unidirectionally toward the heart.

8. The _____ duct drains into the left subclavian vein.

9. The _____ lymph nodes are found clustered in the area of the armpit.

10. _____ lymphocytes are those primarily responsible for distinguishing between normal cells and infected/abnormal (cancer) cells.

11. Lymph nodes have more _____ vessels entering into them than _____ vessels exiting them, which slows flow through the node and allows time for the lymph to be acted upon and filtered.

12. The abbreviation for lymphatic tissue associated with the mucus membranes of the body is _____.

Essay

1. Compare and contrast lymphatic circulation with cardiovascular circulation.

2. Describe the function of the thymus gland.

3. While the spleen is certainly considered a lymphatic organ, discuss some reasons why it is better suited for cardiovascular function.

Respiratory System

8

LEARNING OBJECTIVES

Upon completion of this chapter, the student should be able to:

- Describe the pathway of air from its entry at the mouth and nose through to the lungs
- Locate and describe the components of the upper respiratory tract, including the larynx
- Identify and describe the anatomy of the larynx
- Locate and describe the components of the lower respiratory tract
- Locate the primary and secondary bronchi associated with the lower respiratory tract
- Describe the gross anatomy of the lungs, including their lobes and fissures
- Describe the relationship of the pleural membranes to the lungs

RESPIRATORY SYSTEM OVERVIEW

It is the role of the respiratory system to supply the body with needed oxygen and eliminate carbon dioxide, a waste product of metabolism, to the atmosphere. Collectively, this process is known as ***respiration*** and consists of four distinct phases: **Pulmonary ventilation** is the movement of air in and out of the respiratory tract. It does not involve gas "exchange," but rather simply the movement of air. ***Inhalation*** is an active process in which the diaphragm and external intercostal muscles contract to expand the thoracic cage, drawing air inward. ***Exhalation***, by contrast, is typically a passive process by which the elastic recoil of the lungs makes the thoracic cage smaller, thereby causing air to flow outward. **External respiration** is the exchange of respiratory gases between the gas (air) in the alveoli and the liquid (blood) in the pulmonary capillaries. Oxygen is "loaded" into the blood and carbon dioxide is "unloaded" to the alveoli. The **transportation of the respiratory gases** (O_2 and CO_2) is accomplished with the help of the systemic and pulmonary circuits of the cardiovascular system. **Internal respiration** is the exchange of respiratory gases between the blood of the systemic capillaries and the interstitial fluid of the tissues. Oxygen is "unloaded" to the tissues while carbon dioxide is "loaded" into the systemic capillaries.

To observe an animated overview gas exchange:
*1. Click on **Clinical Animations**; Select "**All**," "**Respiratory**," and "**All**" from the associated drop down menus.*
*2. Click "**Search**."*
*3. Find the animation titled **Gas Exchange**.*

 Gas Exchange

 Lungs

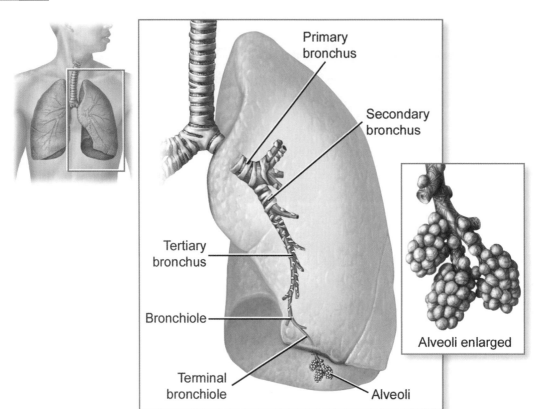

LAB ACTIVITY 8.1

Upper Respiratory System

The upper respiratory system includes those structures that carry air from either the nose or mouth down to and including the larynx. Air is either inhaled through the **nostrils (*nares*)** of the nose into the **nasal cavity** or through the mouth into the **oral cavity**. The nasal and oral cavities are separated by the palate and terminate posteriorly in the region of the pharynx. The anterior aspect of the palate is called the **hard palate** and is made from the union of the two maxillae and palatine bones. The posterior aspect is known as the **soft palate** and consists mostly of muscle fibers enclosed in a mucus membrane. When swallowing, the soft palate closes off the nasal cavity from the oral cavity. The nasal cavity contains three pairs of *nasal conchae*, or **turbinates**. The **superior** and **middle** nasal conchae are part of the ethmoid bone while **the inferior nasal conchae** are individual bones. The conchae are covered by a ciliated mucus membrane and serve to increase the surface area of the nasal cavity, thereby warming, humidifying, and filtering inspired air.

Whether you breathe through the nose or through the mouth, air ultimately enters the region of the **pharynx**, or throat. The region above the palate is known as the **nasopharynx,** which serves as a passageway for air only. Within the nasopharynx may be found the **pharyngeal tonsils,** which are often referred to as ***adenoids***. Also found within the nasopharynx are the openings of the **pharyngotympanic (auditory) tubes**. These passageways serve to equalize the pressure within the middle ear cavity with that of atmospheric air.

CLINICAL APPLICATIONS

Otitis media is an infection of the middle ear cavity most commonly observed in younger children. Because of the proximity of the middle ear to the nasopharynx via the auditory tubes, conditions such as strep throat frequently lead to ear infections in children with immature immune systems.

All of us have experienced the sensation of our ears "popping" at one time or another while driving up a big hill, flying in an airplane, or even when suffering with the common cold. Pressure changes and mucus obstruction can cause the auditory tubes to collapse, creating a vacuum in the middle ear. This vacuum prevents the eardrum from vibrating normally and often causes us to hear muffled sounds. Activities such as swallowing and yawning activate the muscles that open the auditory tubes and allow the air pressure to be restored to normal on either side of the eardrum. That is why it is a good idea to chew gum (or give babies a bottle) when taking off and landing in an airplane. Chewing gum and drinking cause us to swallow more frequently and lessens the chance of our ears "popping," causing that uncomfortable, muffled sensation for the entire flight.

The oral cavity contains the **palatine tonsils** within a pair of folds known as *fauces*. Whether we breathe through the nose or through the mouth, most inspired air comes in contact with tonsils, serving as an important "immunity" role of the respiratory system. Posteriorly, the oral cavity opens into the **oropharynx,** which extends from the soft palate inferiorly to the epiglottis. The **epiglottis** is located within the larynx and is responsible for routing air into the trachea or food into the esophagus. The final division of the throat, behind the epiglottis, is known as the **laryngopharynx**. Both the oropharynx and laryngopharynx are common passageways for air and food.

Identify and label the features of the nasal and oral cavities, and the three divisions of the pharynx in the following figure. To view the image in AIA, go to

 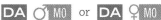 or

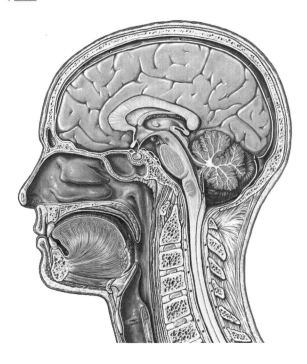

LAB ACTIVITY 8.2

The Larynx

The **larynx** is a collection of both paired and unpaired cartilages collectively known as the "*voicebox*." The largest of these cartilages is the single **thyroid cartilage**. The superior aspect of the thyroid cartilage has a protrusion called the **laryngeal prominence**, or more commonly, the Adam's apple. Inferior to the thyroid cartilage is the single, ring-shaped **cricoid cartilage,** which is smaller from the anterior view and expands posteriorly. Attached to the posterior aspect of the cricoid cartilage are the paired **arytenoid cartilages,** which attach to a set of mucosa-covered folds known as **true vocal cords**. The vibration of these cords, as the name suggests, is responsible for speech. Between the vocal cords is a space leading to the windpipe known as the **glottis**. The **epiglottis** is a flap-like, single cartilage that sits above the glottis and is responsible for routing air and food. While swallowing, the larynx rises to meet the epiglottis, thereby pushing food posteriorly into the esophagus. When breathing, the epiglottis remains upright, allowing air to pass through the glottis into the windpipe. When food or drink goes "down the wrong pipe" it actually enters the larynx, which then initiates a powerful cough reflex in an effort to expel the contents.

Identify and label the hyoid bone, the trachea, and the cartilages of the larynx in the following figures. To locate the images in AIA:

1. *Click on **Atlas Anatomy**; Select "**Head and Neck**," "**Respiratory**," "**Anterior**," and "**Illustration**" from the associated drop down menus.*
2. *Click "**Search**."*
3. *Find the image titled **Laryngeal Muscles (Ant)**.*

AA Laryngeal Muscles (Ant)   **AA** Laryngeal Muscles (Post) 1

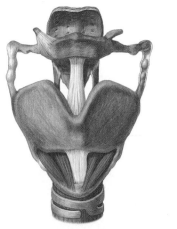 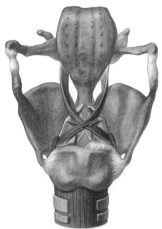

1. *Click on **Atlas Anatomy**; Select "**Head and Neck**," "**Respiratory**," "**Posterior**," and "**Illustration**" from the associated drop down menus.*
2. *Click "**Search**."*
3. *Find the image titled **Laryngeal Muscles (Post) 1**.*

LAB ACTIVITY 8.3

Lower Respiratory System

The **trachea**, or windpipe, extends from the inferior aspect of the larynx downward to the approximate level of the fifth thoracic vertebra before it bifurcates into left and right primary bronchi. The trachea consists of a series of "C"-shaped cartilage rings with the open aspect facing to the posterior. This allows the esophagus to encroach into the tracheal space when swallowing a bolus of food. The **primary (main) bronchi** emerge from the bifurcation point of the trachea known as the *carina*. There is a primary bronchus for each lung; however, the right main bronchus presents as wider, shorter, and more vertical than the left, making it more likely for aspirated objects to get lodged in the right side. The primary bronchi then split into **secondary bronchi** (one for each lobe of the lung), which divide into **tertiary bronchi** (to each bronchopulmonary segment). Branching continues in this manner until eventually they terminate in small **bronchioles**. As the air passages get smaller and smaller they continue to have less cartilage within their walls and gain more smooth muscle. The respiratory bronchioles feed into **alveolar ducts** that terminate in **alveolar sacs** consisting of thousands of tiny air sacs called **alveoli**. Alveoli share a fused basement membrane with respiratory capillaries and allow for external respiration.

Identify and label the trachea, carina, and primary and secondary bronchi in the following figure. To view the image in AIA, go to

   or A252

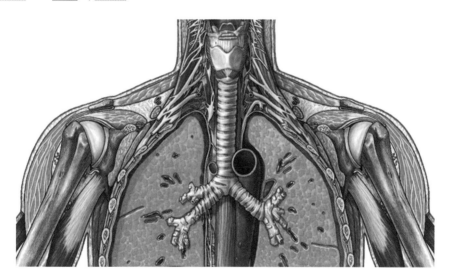

For a closer look at the bronchial tree up to the tertiary bronchi view the following figure. To locate the image in AIA:

1. *Click on **Atlas Anatomy**; Select "**Thorax**," "**Respiratory**," "**Anterior**," and "**Illustration**" from the associated drop down menus.*
2. *Click "**Search**."*
3. *Find the image titled **Bronchial Tree (Ant)**.*

AA | Bronchial Tree (Ant)

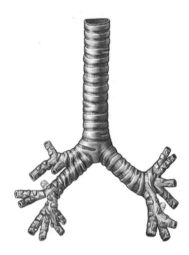

CLINICAL APPLICATIONS

Asthma is a common respiratory disorder characterized by inflammation of the bronchioles and an accompanying increase in mucus production. It is not a disease associated with gas exchange but rather with the movement of air into and out of the lungs, or **ventilation**. When an asthma attack occurs, the muscles surrounding the smaller bronchioles become tight and the lining of the airways swell. This narrowing of the airway leads to wheezing, shortness of breath, chest tightness, and coughing. It is estimated that as many as 1 in 10 children and 1 in 12 adults suffer with some degree of asthma (*Centers for Disease Control and Prevention, Vital Signs, May 2011*). Common asthma triggers include many of the same triggers seen in allergies: animal dander, dust, pollen, cigarette smoke, etc. Asthma may also be induced with stress, exercise (*exercise-induced asthma*), or even a change in the weather. There is no known cure for asthma but symptoms do sometimes improve over time. Preventive measures should include the monitoring of one's environment to minimize exposure to known triggers. Medications such as bronchiole dilators (to open the airways) and inhaled corticosteroids (to reduce inflammation) are commonly prescribed for both the prevention and treatment of asthma attacks. It is important for patients to consult with their health care provider to ensure the treatment they are using is most appropriate for their specific condition.

To view some images of asthma and compare normal versus inflamed bronchioles in AIA:

1. *Click on Clinical Illustrations; Select "**Thorax**," "**Respiratory**," "**All**," "**All**," and "**Pulmonary Medicine**" from the associated drop down menus.*
2. *Click "**Search**."*
3. *Find the corresponding images.*

LAB ACTIVITY 8.4

Gross Anatomy of the Lungs

The paired lungs occupy the majority of the thoracic cavity, each enclosed within its own pleural cavity. The **visceral pleura** is the inner layer intimately associated with the surface of the lung. The **parietal pleura** is adhered to the inner surface of the rib cage and the superior aspect of the diaphragm. The two layers are separated by a potential space, the ***pleural cavity***, which is filled with serous fluid and allows them to easily slide past one another during ventilation. The lungs are roughly triangular shaped with the narrow **apex** located deep to the clavicle and the broader **base** resting inferiorly against the diaphragm. The right lung has three lobes with the **horizontal fissure** separating the **superior** and **middle** lobes and the **oblique fissure** separating the middle and **inferior lobes**. The left lung has a recessed area, the ***cardiac notch***, on its medial aspect to provide room for the heart. It contains only a **superior** and **inferior lobe**, separated by the **oblique fissure**.

Identify and label the lobes, fissures, and features of the lungs in the following figure. To view the image in AIA, go to

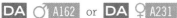

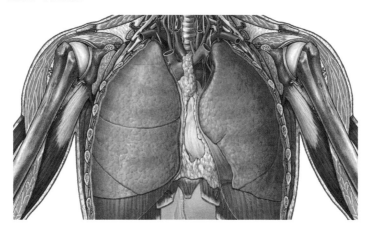

CLINICAL APPLICATIONS

Emphysema is one of the most common respiratory disorders and is often associated with a history of chronic bronchitis. Bronchitis and emphysema are the two main forms of COPD, or chronic obstructive pulmonary disease. Smoking is the leading cause of emphysema and the more a person smokes, the more likely he or she is to develop COPD. Other risk factors include exposure to secondhand smoke, pollution, and occupational exposure to certain fumes in the workplace. Unlike asthma, emphysema is not a disease associated with ***ventilation*** (the movement of air) but rather with gas exchange between the alveoli and blood (***external respiration***). Emphysema causes the destruction of alveolar walls, effectively reducing the size of the respiratory membrane. Emphysema makes it feel like it is hard to catch your breath. The inability to exchange oxygen and carbon dioxide between the lungs and blood often keeps blood oxygen levels lower than normal. There is no known cure for emphysema and symptoms often tend to get worse over time. The single, most important way to avoid accelerated progression of the disease is to quit smoking. Medications such as inhaled corticosteroids to reduce lung inflammation are sometimes prescribed for the treatment of emphysema. Oxygen therapy may also be necessary to increase the concentration of oxygen entering the lungs, thereby increasing oxygen loading into the blood.

To view some images of COPD and compare normal versus damaged alveoli in AIA:
1. *Click on Clinical Illustrations; Select "**Thorax**," "**Respiratory**," "**All**," "**All**," and "**Pulmonary Medicine**" from the associated drop down menus.*
2. *Click "**Search**."*
3. *Find the corresponding images.*

*For a unique interactive experience and a different view of the lower respiratory tract, including the lungs, click on the **3D Anatomy** icon and then select **3D Lungs**.*

3D Lungs

From there you are able to manipulate a three-dimensional recreation by rotating it, moving it, zooming in and out, and even experience cut-away views.

RESPIRATORY SYSTEM REVIEW EXERCISES

Matching

_____ **1.** Internal respiration

_____ **2.** Ventilation

_____ **3.** Trachea

_____ **4.** Adenoids

_____ **5.** Laryngeal prominence

_____ **6.** Secondary bronchi

_____ **7.** External respiration

_____ **8.** Alveoli

_____ **9.** Larynx

_____ **10.** Nasal conchae

a. pharyngeal tonsils

b. gas exchange between blood and tissues

c. turbinates

d. the air sacs of the lungs

e. voicebox

f. gas exchange between blood and air

g. main air supply to each lobe of lungs

h. windpipe

i. the movement of air into and out of the lungs

j. Adam's apple

Labeling

Draw your own lines and then label the following features on the diagram.

a. Auditory tube

b. Epiglottis

c. Nasal conchae

d. Uvula

e. Oropharynx

f. Nostril

g. Hard palate

h. Trachea

i. Pharyngeal tonsil

j. Thyroid cartilage

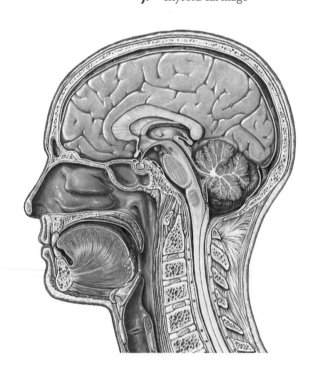

Draw your own lines and then label the following features on the diagram.

    a. Cricoid cartilage

    b. Epiglottis   **e.** Hyoid bone

    c. Vocal cords   **f.** Trachea

    d. Thyroid cartilage   **g.** Arytenoid cartilage

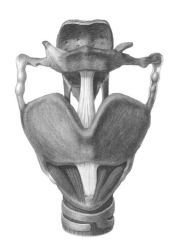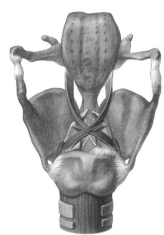

Fill in the Blank/Short Answer

1. The paired cartilages of the larynx are the ＿＿＿＿＿＿＿＿ cartilages.

2. The ＿＿＿＿＿＿＿ primary bronchus is wider, shorter, and more vertical.

3. There are ＿＿＿＿＿＿＿＿ secondary bronchi in the left lung and ＿＿＿＿＿＿＿＿ in the right.

4. The flap-like cartilage that is responsible for routing air and food is the ＿＿＿＿＿＿＿ .

5. The ＿＿＿＿＿＿＿ of the lung is deep to the clavicle while the ＿＿＿＿＿＿＿ of the lung rests on the diaphragm.

6. The division of the throat reserved for air only is the ＿＿＿＿＿＿＿ .

7. The serous membrane attached to the surface of the lung is the ＿＿＿＿＿＿＿.

8. The opening between the vocal cords is the ＿＿＿＿＿＿＿.

9. The ＿＿＿＿＿＿＿ tonsils are found between the fauces of the oral cavity.

10. The hard palate is made from the union of the two anterior ＿＿＿＿＿＿＿ bones and two posterior ＿＿＿＿＿＿＿ bones.

11. The bifurcation of the trachea is known as the ＿＿＿＿＿＿＿.

12. The active phase of ventilation is called ＿＿＿＿＿＿＿ while the passive phase is called ＿＿＿＿＿＿＿.

13. The ＿＿＿＿＿＿＿ lung houses the horizontal fissure.

Essay

1. Describe the four unique events that are collectively called pulmonary respiration.

2. Trace the flow of air from outside the body to the alveoli of the lungs.

3. Briefly discuss the immune function and air "conditioning" mechanism of the respiratory system.

Digestive System

9

Upon completion of this chapter, the student should be able to:

- Locate and identify the organs (and their features) that contribute to the alimentary canal
- Locate and identify the accessory organs (and their features) of the digestive system
- Provide examples of functions for the organs of the digestive system
- Identify the organs and their secretions that contribute to the chemical digestion of macronutrients
- Locate and identify the duct system of the liver, gall bladder, and pancreas
- Be familiar with some of the more common pathological conditions of the digestive system

DIGESTIVE SYSTEM OVERVIEW

Digestion is the process by which we take the food that we eat and transform it into absorbable nutrients that our body needs to perform its seemingly endless list of physiological processes. The digestive system is composed of the **gastrointestinal (GI) tract** or **alimentary canal** (the tube through which the food actually passes) and **accessory organs,** which provide secretions to aid in the digestive process.

Digestion begins with the placing of food into the mouth or **ingestion**. **Propulsion** is the process by which food is moved along the GI Tract. *Peristalsis* is the smooth muscle action that moves food from one organ to the next while *segmentation* is responsible for the mixing or churning of food by smooth muscle as it moves along the GI tract. **Mechanical digestion** occurs with the help of the teeth, the churning action of the stomach, and segmentation in the intestines as larger pieces of ingested food are broken down into smaller more manageable pieces. **Chemical digestion** follows as macronutrients are broken down into their smaller building blocks with the help of enzyme-containing secretions. **Absorption** happens when the digested end products are transported from the lumen of the GI tract into the blood or lymph. Finally, **defecation** is the elimination of indigestible waste products from the GI tract via the rectum and anus in the form of feces.

LAB ACTIVITY 9.1

Head and Neck

Humans form two sets of teeth in their lifetime. The first set of teeth is temporary and begins to emerge around six months of age. A full set of 20 **temporary** teeth (primary, deciduous, or milk teeth) is usually formed by two years of age. As the deciduous teeth begin to loosen and fall out, typically between the ages of 6 and 12, they are replaced by a full set of 32 secondary or **permanent** teeth. Teeth are classified as incisors, cuspids (canines), bicuspids (premolars), and molars.

Identify and label the secondary dentition in the following figure. To locate the image in AIA:
1. *Click on* **Clinical Illustrations**; *Select* **"Head and Neck," "Digestive," "Superior," "Illustration,"** *and* *"Dentistry" from the associated drop down menus.*
2. *Click "***Search.***"*
3. *Find the image titled* **Dental Anatomy***.*

CI | Dental Anatomy |

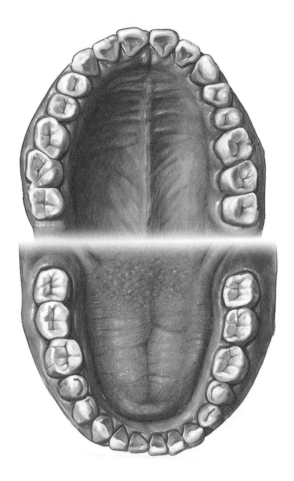

LAB ACTIVITY 9.2

Chemical digestion begins in the mouth with the secretion of saliva by three pairs of salivary glands that open into the oral cavity (**parotid, submandibular, sublingual**). Saliva contains the enzyme **amylase,** which initiates the digestion of carbohydrates into their component monosaccharide building blocks.

Identify and label the three salivary glands in the following figures. To locate the image in AIA:
1. *Click on **Clinical Illustrations**; Select "**Head and Neck**," "**Digestive**," "**Lateral**," "**Illustration**," and "Gastroenterology" from the associated drop down menus.*
2. *Click "**Search**."*
3. *Find the image titled **Head and Neck Glands**.*

CI Head and Neck Glands

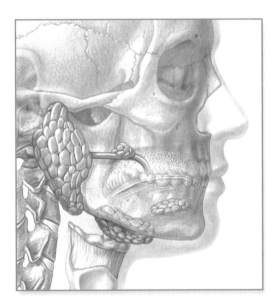

To view the image below in AIA, go to

 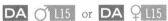 or

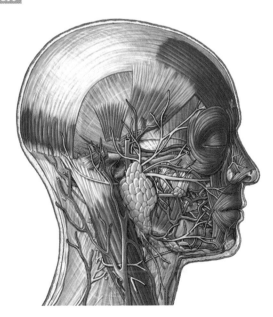

To view the image below in AIA, go to

 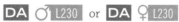 or

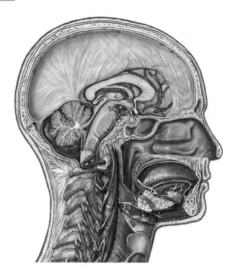

 LAB ACTIVITY 9.3

The tongue is located in the oral cavity. The surface of the tongue is roughened by the presence of various bumps or **papillae**. Some papillae contain taste buds (chemoreceptors) while others simply provide friction. Taste buds are located on **fungiform, circumvallate**, and **foliate** papillae while the numerous small **filiform** papillae act to provide roughness and friction to the tongue.

Identify and label the four types of papillae in the figure below. To locate the image in AIA:
1. *Click on* **Atlas Anatomy**; *Select* "**Head and Neck**," "**Digestive**," "**Superior**," *and* "**Illustration**" *from the associated drop down menus.*
2. *Click* "**Search**."
3. *Find the image titled* **Surface of Tongue (Dorsal)**.

AA Surface of Tongue (Dorsal)

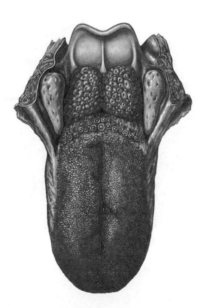

The oral cavity is separated from the nasal cavity by the **hard palate** and the **soft palate**. The **uvula** is located at the posterior aspect of the soft palate. Once the ingested food is chewed (masticated) and mixed with saliva, it becomes a bolus, which is then pushed back into the **pharynx** and swallowed. The uvula serves to block off the nasal cavity from the oral cavity during this process to ensure the bolus gets pushed inferiorly toward the **esophagus**.

Identify and label the hard palate, soft palate, uvula, tongue, pharynx, and esophagus in the figure below. To view the image in AIA, go to

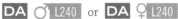 or

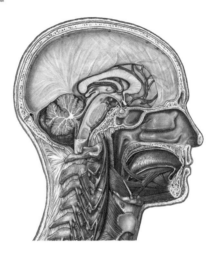

The esophagus delivers the bolus of food from the pharynx, through the diaphragm, into the abdominal cavity to connect to the **stomach** at the **lower esophageal (cardiac) sphincter**. The stomach is highly acidic (pH of approximately 2.0) and is the initial site of protein digestion. The production of hydrochloric acid is necessary to activate pepsinogen to pepsin, which is the active protein digesting enzyme. The partially digested foodstuff at this stage is now referred to as "chyme."

CLINICAL APPLICATIONS

On occasion, a weak cardiac sphincter may allow the acidic content of the stomach to flow upward into the esophagus causing a pain commonly referred to as *heartburn* or *GERD (gastroesophageal reflux disease)*. Another common cause of heartburn occurs when the superior aspect of the stomach protrudes upward through the diaphragm causing a condition called **hiatal hernia**.

To view the image in AIA:
1. *Click on Clinical Illustrations; Select "**Abdomen**," "**Digestive**," "**Anterior**," "**Illustration**," and "**Gastroenterolgy**" from the associated drop down menus.*
2. *Click "**Search**."*
3. *Find the image titled **Hiatal Hernia - Sectional View**.*

 Hiatal Hernia

ABDOMEN

 LAB ACTIVITY 9.5

The stomach has four major regions: the **cardiac** region connects to the esophagus, the **fundus** is the superior portion, the **body** is the midportion, and the **pylorus** connects the stomach to the small intestine. The empty stomach causes the stomach to "ripple" into ridges called **rugae** as it assumes a smaller shape. The **lesser omentum** is a double layered peritoneum that connects the concave medial surface of the stomach (**lesser curvature**) to the **liver** while the **greater omentum** drapes from the convex lateral surface (**greater curvature**) to cover the abdominal organs like an apron.

Identify and label the esophagus, the regions of the stomach, liver, gall bladder, lesser omentum, greater omentum, and transverse colon in the figures below. To locate the image in AIA:

*1. Click on **Atlas Anatomy**; Select "**Abdomen**," "**Digestive**," "**Anterior**," and "**Illustration**" from the associated drop down menus.*
*2. Click "**Search**."*
*3. Find the image titled **Stomach 1**.*

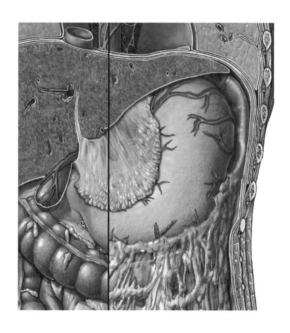

To view the image below in AIA, go to

 or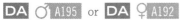

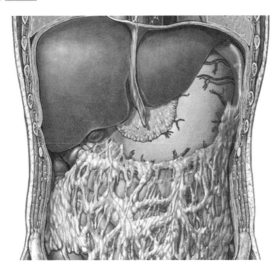

*Try to compare as many features as you can identify from the illustrations in Lab activity 9.5 to the Cadaver Photograph in the image below.

To locate the image in AIA:
1. *Click on* **Atlas Anatomy***; Select* "**Abdomen**," "**Digestive**," "**Anterior**," *and* "**Cadaver Photo**" *from the associated drop down menus.*
2. *Click* "**Search***.*"
3. *Find the image titled* **Stomach & Spleen (Ant) 2***.*

AA Stomach & Spleen (Ant) 2

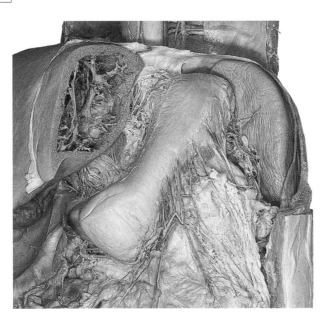

LAB ACTIVITY 9.6

The rugae may be visualized in the following images. To locate the image in AIA:
1. *Click on **Atlas Anatomy**; Select "**Abdomen**," "**Digestive**," "**Anterior**," and "**Illustration**" from the associated drop down menus.*
2. *Click "**Search**."*
3. *Find the image titled **Stomach & Spleen (Ant) 1**.*

AA Stomach & Spleen (Ant) 1

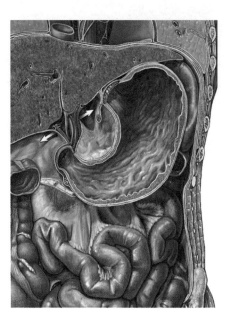

To view the following image in AIA, go to

  or

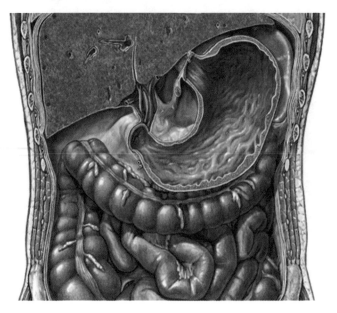

LAB ACTIVITY 9.7

The **small intestine** consists of three subdivisions: **duodenum**, **jejunum**, and **ileum**. The proximal portion, the **duodenum**, is only 10 inches long and connects to the pylorus of the stomach at the **pyloric sphincter**. Ducts from the **liver**, **gall bladder**, and **pancreas** deliver bile and digestive enzymes to the duodenum to initiate lipid digestion and complete the digestion of carbohydrates, proteins, and nucleic acids. Bile is necessary to emulsify, or prepare, fats for digestion by lipase enzymes. **Bile** is produced by the liver and stored in the gall bladder. The presence of fatty chyme in the duodenum signals the liver to deliver bile through the **right and left hepatic ducts** to the **common hepatic duct** where it joins with the **cystic duct** from the gall bladder to form the **common bile duct**. The common bile duct then merges with the **main pancreatic duct,** which is carrying alkaline, enzyme-rich pancreatic juice to enter the duodenum at the **hepatopancreatic ampulla/ papilla**. Distal to the duodenum, the small intestine continues as the 6-foot-long jejunum, which then connects to the terminal part of the small intestine, the 10-foot-long section known as the ileum. The movement of foodstuffs along the entire alimentary canal, including the small intestine is known as **peristalsis**.

Identify and label the various ducts associated with the liver, gall bladder, and pancreas on the following figures. Also notice and label the esophagus; pyloric sphincter; gall bladder; the head, body, and tail of the pancreas; and the right/left lobes of the liver. To locate the image in AIA:
1. *Click on **Atlas Anatomy**; Select "**Abdomen**," "**Digestive**," "**Anterior**," and "**Illustration**" from the associated drop down menus.*
2. *Click "**Search**."*
3. *Find the image titled **Pancreatic & Bile Ducts 1**.*

AA | Pancreatic & Bile Ducts 1

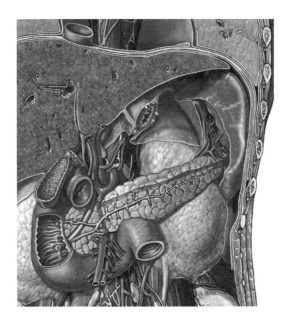

To view the image below in AIA, go to

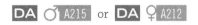

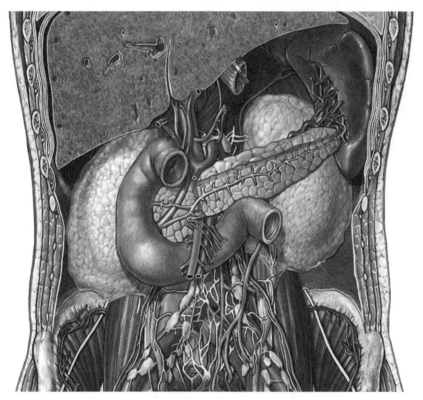

To visualize the process of peristalsis:
1. *Click on **Clinical Animations**; Select "**All**," "**Digestive**," and "**All**" from the associated drop down menus.*
2. *Click "**Search**."*
3. *Find the animation titled **Peristalsis**.*

'Try to compare as many features as you can identify from the illustrations in Lab Activity 9.7 to the Cadaver Photograph in the image below.

To locate the image in AIA:
1. *Click on* **Atlas Anatomy***; Select* "**Abdomen**," "**Digestive**," "**Anterior**," *and* "**Cadaver Photo**" *from the associated drop down menus.*
2. *Click "***Search***."*
3. *Find the image titled* **Stomach & Spleen (Ant) 2***.*

AA Pancreas & Spleen (Ant)

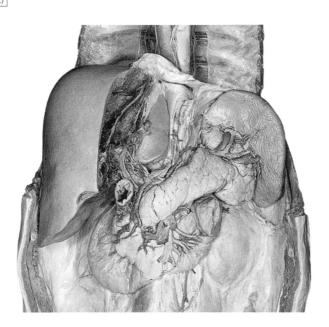

To view radiographic images of the biliary duct system as well as the stomach and small intestine:
1. *Click on* **Atlas Anatomy***; Select "***Abdomen***," "***Digestive***," "***Anterior***," and "***Radiograph***" from the associated drop down menus.*
2. *Click "***Search***."*
3. *Find the images titled* **Cholangiopancreatogram (Ant)** *and* **Barium in Small Bowel***.*

AA Cholangiopancreatogram (Ant)   **AA** Barium in Small Bowel

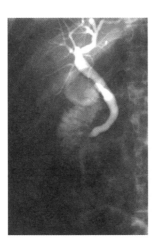 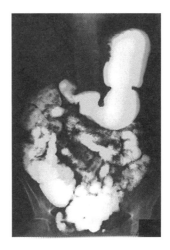

CLINICAL APPLICATIONS

On occasion, bile salts and cholesterol within the gall bladder collect into hard masses commonly known as gallstones contributing to a condition known as **cholelithiasis**. If these gall stones aggregate in the duct system it is then referred to as **choledocholithiasis**.

To view images of gall stones and choledocholithiasis on AIA:
1. Click on *Clinical Illustrations*; Select *"Abdomen," "Digestive," "Anterior," "Illustration,"* and *"Gastroenterology"* from the associated drop down menus.
2. Click *"Search."*
3. Find the images titled Gallstone, *Bile Pathway*, and *Choledocholithiasis*.

CI | Gall Stone   **CI** | Bile Pathway

CI | Choledocholithiasis

 LAB ACTIVITY 9.8

The **liver** is the largest gland in the body and has numerous metabolic and regulatory roles. The liver is located on the right side of the abdominal cavity, resting directly below the **diaphragm** and suspended by the **falciform ligament**. The four lobes of the liver are the right, left, caudate, and quadrate lobes. Its main digestive function is the production of bile as discussed earlier.

Identify and label the right and left lobes of the liver, the diaphragm, and the falciform ligament from the figure below. To view the image below in AIA, go to

DA ♂ A196 or **DA** ♀ A193

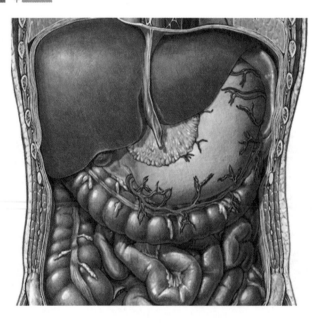

LAB ACTIVITY 9.9

You may also view all four lobes of the liver from the additional image below. To locate the image in AIA:
1. *Click on **Atlas Anatomy**; Select "**Abdomen**," "**Digestive**," "**Inferior**," and "**Illustration**" from the associated drop down menus.*
2. *Click "**Search**."*
3. *Find the image titled **Liver (Inf).***

AA Liver (Inf)

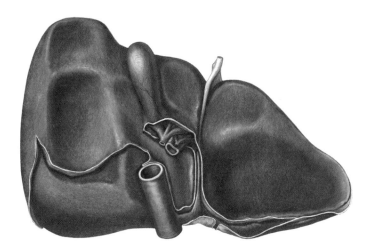

CLINICAL APPLICATIONS

A chronic disease causing damage to liver tissue, scarring of the liver, and a progressive decrease in liver function is a condition known as **cirrhosis**. The most common cause of cirrhosis is excessive alcohol use.

To view an image of liver cirrhosis in AIA:
1. *Click on Clinical Illustrations; Select "**Abdomen**," "**Digestive**," "**Anterior**," "**Illustration**," and "**Gastroenterology**" from the associated drop down menus.*
2. *Click "**Search**."*
3. *Find the image titled **Cirrhosis of the Liver**.*

CI Cirrhosis of the Liver

LAB ACTIVITY 9.10

The **large intestine (colon)** connects proximally to the small intestine at the **ileocecal junction** and terminates distally at the **rectum**. The large intestine is involved in feces formation and is the major site of water absorption. Normal flora bacteria within the large intestine contribute to the production of vitamins such as vitamin K and vitamin B_{12}. Externally, the visual appearance of the large intestine presents as a longitudinal collection of sac-like structures known as "**haustra**." Additionally, three distinct longitudinal bands of smooth muscle, **taenia coli**, can be visualized running along the entire length of the large intestine. The initial segment of the colon is known as the **cecum** where the **vermiform appendix** (a lymphatic structure) is attached. The **ascending colon** travels up the right side of the abdominal cavity before making a turn at the **right colic (hepatic) flexure**. The **transverse colon** travels across the abdominal cavity before turning downward at the **left colic (splenic)** flexure to become the **descending colon,** which then becomes the "S-shaped" **sigmoid colon** as it enters the pelvis to then join into the rectum.

Identify and label the divisions of the large intestine as well as the vermiform appendix, ileum, ileocecal junction, and taenia coli from the figure below. To locate the image in AIA:
1. *Click on* ***Atlas Anatomy****; Select "****Abdomen****," "****Digestive****," "****Anterior****," and "****Illustration****," from the associated drop down menus.*
2. *Click "****Search****."*
3. *Find the image titled* ***Large Intestine In Situ****.*

AA | Large Intestine In Situ

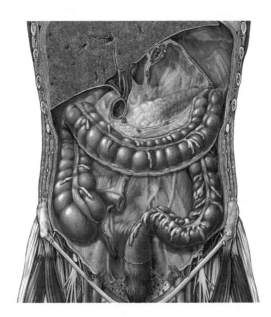

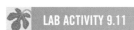 **LAB ACTIVITY 9.11**

Major divisions of the large intestine may also be visualized in the figure below. To view the image below in AIA, go to

  or 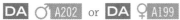 A199

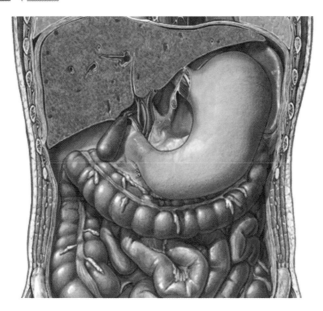

To view a radiographic image of the large bowel:
1. *Click on **Atlas Anatomy**; Select "**Abdomen**," "**Digestive**," "**Anterior**," and "**Radiograph**" from the associated drop down menus.*
2. *Click "**Search**."*
3. *Find the image titled **Barium in Large Bowel**.*

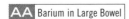
Barium in Large Bowel

CLINICAL APPLICATIONS

A colonoscopy is a procedure that allows the physician to insert a flexible camera into the large intestine to visually inspect the mucosal surface. Ulcerative colitis and Chrohn disease are two examples of **inflammatory bowel disease**.

To view corresponding images in AIA:
1. *Click on Clinical Illustrations; Select "**Abdomen**," "**Digestive**," "**Anterior**," "**Illustration**," and "**Gastroenterology**" from the associated drop down menus.*
2. *Click "**Search**."*
3. *Find the images titled **Colonoscopy** and **Inflammatory Bowel Disease**.*

CI Colonoscopy   CI Inflammatory Bowel Disease

Another common reason for a colonoscopy is to screen for colon cancer.
1. *Click on Clinical Illustrations; Select "**Abdomen**," "**Digestive**," "**Anterior**," "**Illustration**," and "**Gastroenterology**" from the associated drop down menus.*
2. *Click "**Search**."*
3. *Find the image titled **Stages of Cancer** to see a representation of the three stages of colon cancer.*

CI Stages of Cancer

In severe cases, it may be necessary to remove the cancerous portion of the colon at which time the patient must collect their feces into a bag attached to an opening in the abdominal wall. This procedure is known as a colostomy.

1. *Click on Clinical Illustrations; Select "**Abdomen**," "**Digestive**," "**Anterior**," "**Illustration**," and "**Gastroenterology**" from the associated drop down menus.*
2. *Click "**Search**."*
3. *Find the image titled **Colostomy** to view this procedure.*

CI Colostomy

PELVIS

LAB ACTIVITY 9.12

The alimentary canal terminates in the **rectum** and **anus**. The rectum receives its contents from the sigmoid colon and then stores the feces and compacts it until it is ready to be eliminated via a process known as **defecation**. Three **transverse folds** in the rectum aid in the separation of flatus (gas) from the feces. At the junction of the rectum and anus small folds of mucosa, **anal columns**, may be visualized. The anus is the final 1.5 inches of the GI tract and is composed of two distinct sphincters: the **internal anal sphincter** is made of smooth muscle and is under involuntary control while the **external anal sphincter** is made of skeletal muscle and is under voluntary control.

Identify and label the rectum with its folds, the anus, anal columns, and the internal and external anal sphincters using the figures below. To locate the image in AIA:
1. *Click on **Atlas Anatomy**; Select "**Pelvis and Perineum**," "**Digestive**," "**Anterior**," and "**Illustration**" from the associated drop down menus.*
2. *Click "**Search**."*
3. *Find the image titled **Frontal Section of Anal Canal**.*

AA | Frontal Section of Anal Canal

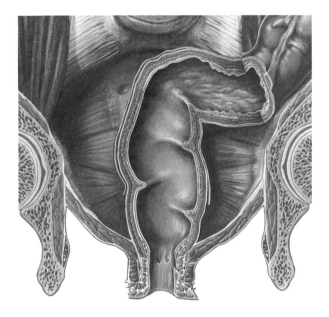

1. *Click on* **Atlas Anatomy**; *Select* "**Pelvis and Perineum**," "**Digestive**," "**Medial**," *and* "**Illustration**" *from the associated drop down menus.*
2. *Click* "**Search**."
3. *Find the image titled* **Sagittal Section of Rectum**.

AA | Sagittal Section of Rectum |

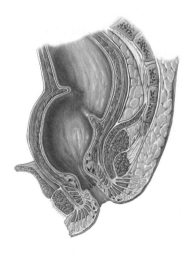

CLINICAL APPLICATIONS

Hemorrhoids are a condition of swollen veins in the anal canal. Hemorrhoids may be internal, external, or both, and are commonly caused by an increase in pressure on the veins in the pelvic and rectal areas. Hemorrhoids may be caused by a variety of issues but are more common during pregnancy and in those individuals who strain excessively during a bowel movement, such as with constipation.

To view an image of hemorrhoids in AIA:
1. *Click on* Clinical Illustrations; *Select* "**Pelvis and Perineum**," "**Digestive**," "**Medial**," "**Illustration**" *and* "**Gastroenterology**" *from the associated drop down menus.*
2. *Click* "**Search**."
3. *Find the image titled* **Hemorrhoids**.

CI | Hemorrhoids |

DIGESTIVE SYSTEM REVIEW EXERCISES

Matching

_____ **1.** Absorption

_____ **2.** Chemical digestion

_____ **3.** Peristalsis

_____ **4.** Defecation

_____ **5.** Ingestion

_____ **6.** Mechanical digestion

_____ **7.** Segmentation

a. the process of breaking down larger pieces of ingested food into smaller ones

b. the elimination of indigestible wastes from the GI tract

c. the mixing/churning of food by smooth muscle as it moves along the GI tract

d. the breakdown of macronutrients by enzymes into their building blocks

e. the movement of digestive end products into the blood or lymph

f. the placement of food into the mouth

g. the smooth muscle action that propels food along the GI tract

Labeling

Draw your own lines and then label the following features on the diagram.

a. Stomach

b. Liver

c. Small intestine

d. Rectum

e. Esophagus

f. Gall bladder

g. Pancreas

h. Large intestine

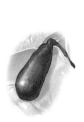
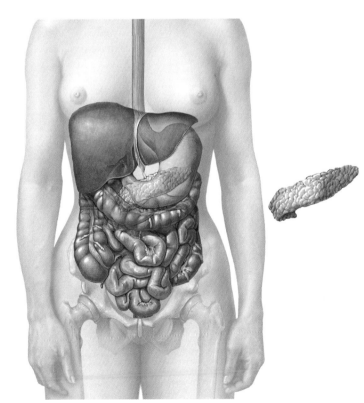

Draw your own lines and then label the following features on the diagram.

a. Pancreas
b. Left lobe of liver
c. Gall bladder
d. Main pancreatic duct
e. Duodenum
f. Cystic duct

g. Hepatopancreatic ampulla/papilla
h. Pyloric sphincter
i. Hepatic duct
j. Common bile duct
k. Right lobe of liver
l. Esophagus

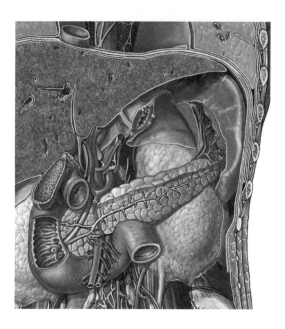

Draw your own lines and then label the following features on the diagram.

a. Vermiform appendix
b. Ileum
c. Pyloric sphincter
d. Haustra
e. Taeniae coli

f. Regions of colon (cecum, ascending colon, hepatic flexure, transverse colon, splenic flexure, descending colon,
sigmoid colon)
g. Rectum

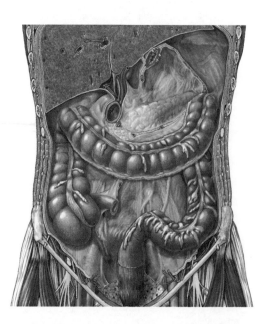

Fill in the Blank/Short Answer

1. The three pairs of salivary glands are the _____, _____, and _____.

2. Bile is produced by the _____, stored in the _____, and is necessary to emulsify _____.

3. Chemical digestion of protein begins in the _____.

4. A complete set of adult dentition contains _____ permanent (secondary) teeth.

5. The primary site of water absorption is the _____.

6. Saliva contains the enzyme _____, which initiates digestion of _____.

7. Dilated (varicose) veins in the anus is a condition known as _____.

8. The organ where the majority of fat digestion occurs is the _____.

9. The _____ anal sphincter is voluntary while the _____ anal sphincter is involuntary.

10. The common bile duct is made from the union of the _____ and the _____.

11. Name the three divisions of the small intestine from proximal to distal. _____, _____, _____.

12. Define "G.E.R.D." and give one possible _____ _____.

13. Which one of the four types of tongue papillae does NOT contain any taste buds? _____.

Essay

1. Describe the sequential order of organs in the alimentary canal from the mouth through the anus.

2. Describe the accessory organs of digestion and indicate the general function of each.

Urinary System

LEARNING OBJECTIVES

Upon completion of this chapter, the student should be able to:

- Locate and describe the organs of the urinary system

- Describe the renal artery and its branches within the kidney

- Describe the internal anatomy of the kidney including structures of the cortex and medulla

- Describe the structure and function of the renal corpuscle

- Describe the pathway of urine (filtrate) through the nephron

- Identify the three openings in the urinary bladder and describe the route of urine

- Locate the female urethra and describe its relationship to other structures of the perineum

- Locate the male urethra with its three distinct regions and describe its dual function as both a urinary and reproductive structure

- Locate the prostate gland and describe its relationship to the male urethra

URINARY SYSTEM OVERVIEW

The urinary system is our body's primary waste disposal system. It is composed of paired **kidneys**, paired **ureters**, and a singular **urinary bladder** and **urethra**. Asleep or awake, the body is constantly undergoing a mind-boggling number of metabolic reactions, which in turn produce a host of different waste products that are transported in the bloodstream. The kidneys serve as the major blood filters of the body, eliminating metabolic wastes in the urine while returning necessary nutrients to the bloodstream. While only one vessel, the renal artery, carries oxygenated, but waste-riddled, blood into the kidney, there are two exit routes from the kidney. The renal vein carries deoxygenated, but cleansed, blood back toward the inferior vena cava while the ureters carry waste-filled plasma (now called urine) toward the bladder for eventual elimination from the body via the urethra.

1. *Click on* **Clinical Illustrations**; *Select* "**Abdomen**," "**Urinary**," "**Anterior**," "**Illustration**," *and* "**Urology**" *from the associated drop down menus.*
2. *Click* "**Search**."
3. *Find the image titled* **Female Urinary Tract.**

CI Female Urinary Tract

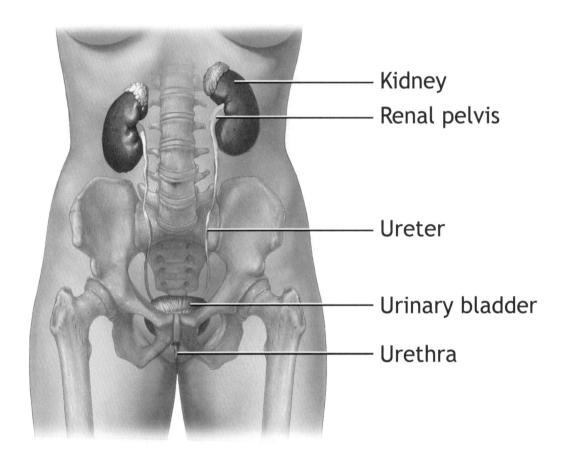

Kidney

Renal pelvis

Ureter

Urinary bladder

Urethra

LAB ACTIVITY 10.1

External Kidney Features

The kidneys are considered *retroperitoneal,* so in order to see them from the anterior aspect the peritoneum must be removed. The kidneys are anchored in place and protected by an outer renal adipose capsule and supporting renal fascia. Resting atop each kidney sits the **suprarenal (adrenal) gland**. On the concave side of the "bean-shaped" kidney may be found the renal *hilum*. The hilum is the area for the renal artery to enter as well as the place for the renal vein and ureter to exit the kidney. Each **ureter** begins proximally at an expanded, funnel-shaped region known as the **renal pelvis** before narrowing and proceeding inferiorly toward the **urinary bladder**.

Identify and label the kidneys, adrenal glands, ureters, renal artery and vein, abdominal aorta, and inferior vena cava in the following figure. To view the image in AIA, go to

 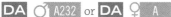

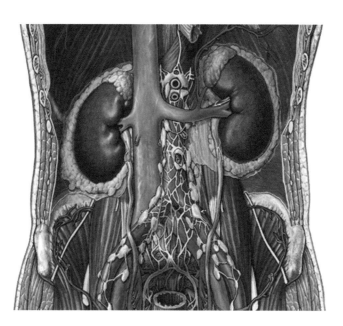

CLINICAL APPLICATIONS

Occasionally, there may be situations where someone is unable to voluntarily control urination, such as when a person is hospitalized or suffers from certain urinary pathologies. In cases such as these, it may be necessary to *catheterize* the individual in order to drain the urinary bladder. A **catheter** is a flexible, hollow tube similar to a soft drinking straw, which is inserted into the urethra from the outside. The urine is then drained and collected into a bag for analysis purposes. A **cystoscopy** is a procedure that allows a physician to view the inside of the bladder for purposes of diagnosis and tissue sample collection (biopsy). Once a urinary catheter is in place a small fiber optic instrument, a *cystoscope*, is inserted through the catheter into the urinary bladder to allow for visual inspection.

To view some images of catheterization and cystoscopy in AIA:
1. *Click on "Clinical Illustrations"; Select "**Pelvis and Perineum**," "**Urinary**," "**All**," "**All**," and "**Urology**" from the associated drop down menus.*
2. *Click "**Search**."*
3. *Find the corresponding images.*

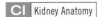 **LAB ACTIVITY 10.2**

Internal Kidney Features

In coronal (frontal) section, the major divisions of the kidneys may be easily identified. The outer, thinner, more lightly colored region is known as the **cortex**. The majority of nephrons (called "*cortical nephrons*") are located in this region. The inner, thicker region is known as the **medulla**. The majority of the medulla is occupied by a number (typically between 7 and 12) of triangular, striated **pyramids**. The base of each pyramid faces the outer cortex while the apex points toward the deeper cup-like receiving areas known as *calyces*. The striated pattern of the pyramids results from the vertical orientation of the **collecting ducts,** which are delivering urine from the nephron toward the calyces. A thin strip of cortical-like tissue known as the **renal column** extends into the medulla separating each pyramid. A pyramid with its cortical tissue above it is known as a lobe of the kidney. Each pyramid empties its urine into a small receiving area known as a **minor calyx**. A few minor calyces will then merge into a larger, **major calyx**. Each kidney contains two or three major calyces, which then merge into the larger, funnel-shaped **renal pelvis,** which will then exit the kidney and transport urine toward the bladder for storage via the ureter.

1. *Click on **Clinical Illustrations**; Select "**Abdomen**," "**Urinary**," "**Anterior**," "**Illustration**," and "**Urology**" from the associated drop down menus.*
2. *Click "**Search**."*
3. *Find the image titled **Kidney Anatomy**.*

CI Kidney Anatomy

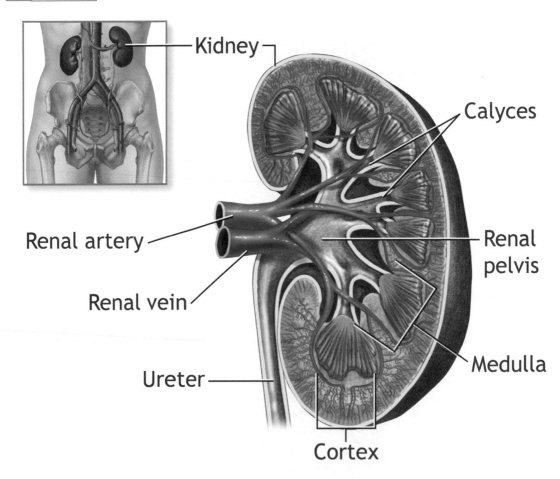

To view a similar image of the inner kidney you may go to **DA** ♂ A240 *or* **DA** ♀ A239 *and label the features listed in this lab activity.*

CLINICAL APPLICATIONS

Kidney stones, or *nephroliths*, are collections of crystals that separate from the urine while in the urinary tract, often accumulating in the calyces and interfering with normal kidney function. Kidney stones are generally composed up of calcium and additional chemicals such as oxalate and phosphate, which are part of a regular diet and may also be found within tissues of the body such as bone and muscle. In extreme cases, the stones may congeal into a large mass known as a *staghorn calculus,* which occupies the calyces as well as the entire renal pelvis. Staghorn calculi may be visualized with standard x-ray procedures and surgical removal is typically necessary to remove these larger stones. Since smaller stones often escape detection with traditional x-ray, a special x-ray known as an **IVP (*intravenous pyelogram*)** involves injecting a radiopaque dye into the patient's vein and then using the x-ray to view the flow of dye through the urinary tract. Smaller stones occasionally dislodge themselves and progress through the remaining organs of the urinary system. In some instance, they make it all the way out of the body to be eliminated in the urine, while in other cases they get stuck along the way. As kidney stones traverse through the ureters they cause an incredible amount of pain, often presenting as low back or flank pain. There may also be noticeable traces of blood in the urine (*hematuria*) as these jagged stones irritate the lining of the passageways along their journey. The intense pain is followed by welcomed relief once the stone makes its way into the much larger diameter bladder, but there is still one more tube to go. To be eliminated from the body, the stone must finally be passed through the urethra, which again is associated with a great deal of discomfort. In cases where large stones are incapable of being passed from the body, a procedure known as *extracorporeal shock wave lithotripsy (ESWL)* may be performed in an effort to break up the stones into smaller, more manageable pieces. ESWL is a form of ultrasound that uses focused sound waves to slough off the outer layers of the stone until they are small enough to be eliminated from the body. Dietary modification, and sometimes medications, may be advised to minimize the risk of recurring kidney stones.

To view some images of catheterization and cystoscopy in AIA:
1. *Click on "Clinical Illustrations"; Select "**Abdomen**," "**Urinary**," "**All**," "**All**," and "**Urology**" from the associated drop down menus.*
2. *Click "**Search**."*
3. *Find the corresponding images.*

LAB ACTIVITY 10.3

Blood Supply to the Kidney

The **abdominal aorta** gives rise to the **renal arteries,** which deliver blood to their respective kidney. As much as 25% of cardiac output flows through the kidneys each minute! Upon entering the kidney at the hilum, the renal artery divides into two or three **segmental arteries**. Each segmental artery then divides into a few **lobar arteries**. The lobar arteries branch into **interlobar arteries,** which ascend toward the cortex along the renal columns. The interlobar arteries give off arching branches called **arcuate arteries,** which are found lying atop of the pyramids. The arcuate arteries give off branches that radiate into the cortex called **interlobular** or **cortical radiate arteries**. The cortical radiate arteries give rise to the many **afferent arterioles,** which supply blood to the capillary networks of the individual nephrons—the *glomeruli* and *peritubular capillaries*. Blood from these capillary plexuses is drained into the **cortical radiate veins**, to the **arcuate veins**, to the **interlobar veins**, and out to the **renal vein** en route to the **inferior vena cava**. There are no named lobar or segmental veins in the kidney.

Identify and label the blood vessels of the kidney in the following figure.

To locate the image in AIA:

1. *Click on **Atlas Anatomy**; Select "**Abdomen**," "**Urinary**," "**Posterior**," and "**Illustration**" from the associated drop down menus.*
2. *Click "**Search**."*
3. *Find the image titled **Renal Arteries**.*

AA | Renal Arteries

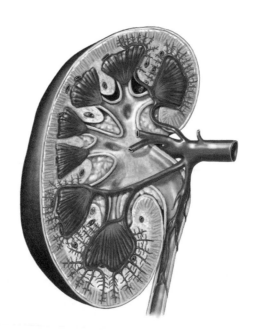

LAB ACTIVITY 10.4

The Renal Corpuscle

The structural and functional unit of the kidney is known as the **nephron**, with each kidney containing as many as one million nephrons apiece. It is the nephron, which is responsible for filtering the blood; separating the metabolic wastes (in the form of urine) from the needed nutrients, which get returned to general circulation. **Filtration** is a passive process that is driven by hydrostatic (blood) pressure. Each nephron is composed of a specialized capillary, called a **glomerulus**, and a **renal tubule**. The part of the renal tubule that encases the glomerulus, receiving the filtrate, is called the **glomerular (Bowman) capsule**. The glomerulus and its respective capsule are collectively known as the **renal corpuscle**. The capillaries are surrounded by specialized cells, called *podocytes*, which have interdigitating, foot-like processes that form filtration slits. Any substances smaller than the space between the filtration slits are capable of leaving circulation and entering into the filtrate. The glomerulus has two unique features that make it specially adapted for filtration. First, they are fenestrated ("containing windows"), which makes them more permeable than other systemic capillaries. Secondly, the glomeruli are both fed and drained by arterioles. The larger diameter afferent arteriole supplies blood to the glomerulus while the smaller diameter efferent arteriole drains the glomerulus. Because the efferent arteriole has a smaller diameter, it allows for a higher hydrostatic pressure within the glomerulus, which is the driving force of glomerular filtration. The *juxtaglomerular apparatus* (**juxtaglomerular cells** within the afferent arteriole and **macula densa cells** within the distal convoluted tubule) assist in regulating what is known as the **glomerular filtration rate (GFR)**.

Identify and label the components of the renal corpuscle in the following figure.
To locate the image in AIA:
1. *Click on **Atlas Anatomy**; Select "**Abdomen**," "**Urinary**," "**Non-standard**," and "**Illustration**" from the associated drop down menus.*
2. *Click "**Search**."*
3. *Find the image titled **Diagram of Renal Glomerulus**.*

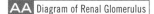

AA Diagram of Renal Glomerulus

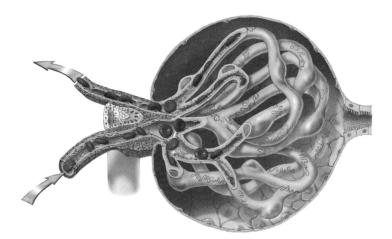

LAB ACTIVITY 10.5

The Renal Tubule

The **renal tubule** is responsible for adjusting the filtrate in order to assure homeostasis. Blood volume, blood pressure, pH, and electrolyte balance are all dependent on the nephron's ability to adjust its contents. The renal tubule is surrounded by a network of capillaries known as **peritubular capillaries**. These capillaries are under low pressure, which makes them specially modified to absorb the contents of the interstitial fluid. Once plasma leaves the glomerulus and enters the **glomerular capsule** as *filtrate* it continues into the **proximal convoluted tubule (PCT)**. The PCT is responsible for returning the majority of filtrate back into circulation via the peritubular capillaries through a process known as tubular reabsorption. From the PCT filtrate enters into the **loop of Henle**. The *thin, descending limb* dives down toward the medulla while the *thick, ascending limb* works its way back toward the cortex. The two limbs are permeable to different substances (water and solutes) along their length, allowing the filtrate to be further modified along its journey. Specialized peritubular capillaries follow the course of the loop of Henle and are known as **vasa recta**. The ascending limb continues into the **distal convoluted tubule (DCT),** which then drains into a **collecting duct**. The DCTs and collecting ducts are more or less impermeable to water or solutes in the absence of hormones. *Aldosterone* increases the permeability of the tubule cells to sodium whereas *antidiuretic hormone* (ADH) allows the nephron to reclaim as much as 95% of the fluid volume of the filtrate in cases of dehydration and hypovolemia. Each collecting duct courses through the pyramids, receiving the DCTs of a number of nephrons along the way, eventually emptying into the calyces.

Identify and label the components of the nephron in the following figure.

To locate the image in AIA:

1. *Click on **Atlas Anatomy**; Select "**Abdomen**," "**Urinary**," "**Anterior**," and "**Illustration**" from the associated drop down menus.*
2. *Click "**Search**."*
3. *Find the image titled **Diagram of Nephron**.*

AA Diagram of Nephron

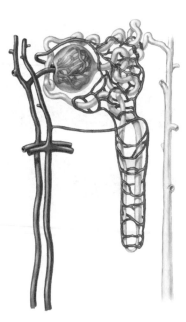

LAB ACTIVITY 10.6

The Bladder and Urethra

Transporting urine from the renal pelvis to the bladder, via peristaltic contractions, are the **ureters**. The ureters enter the urinary bladder toward the inferior, posterolateral wall. The bladder is a thick, muscular organ designed as a holding tank capable of storing as much as 500 mL (approximately one pint) or so of urine. In the midsagittal view of the female pelvis, you can see how the urinary bladder is sandwiched between the uterus to the posterior and the pubic symphysis to the anterior. In a pregnant female, it is easy to see how there is little room for the bladder to expand, which helps account for the increased frequency of urination during pregnancy. In the floor of the bladder is found the singular opening for the **urethra**. The three openings in the bladder—one for each ureter plus the urethra, form a triangular area known as the ***trigone***. The trigone is clinically important for it is a frequent site of urinary tract infections. Two urinary sphincters surround the origin of the urethra: the smooth muscle, involuntarily controlled **internal urethral sphincter,** and the skeletal muscle, voluntarily controlled **external urethral sphincter**.

The female **urethra** is strictly a urinary system passageway and averages just over 1.5 inches in length, exiting the body just anterior to the vaginal orifice. Because of its short length and proximity to the anus, improper toiletry habits can introduce bacteria into the urethra, contributing to higher incidences of urinary tract infections in women as compared to men. The male urethra is longer than the females, averaging 7.5 inches or so in length and serves as both a urinary and reproductive system passageway. As the male urethra exits the bladder, it courses through the chestnut-sized prostate gland as the **prostatic urethra**. As the urethra continues through the muscles of the urogenital diaphragm for a short time it is known as the **membranous urethra**. Upon entering the corpus spongiosum of the penis, it then becomes the **penile (spongy) urethra**. The spongy urethra accounts for as much as 75% of the entire urethral length. Merging with the prostatic urethra is the ejaculatory duct, containing a mixture of sperm and accessory gland secretions. At the time of ejaculation, the urethral sphincters at the base of the bladder are forced closed as the urethra now serves as a reproductive conduit.

CLINICAL APPLICATIONS

In cases of **benign prostatic hypertrophy (BPH),** it may be incredibly difficult for a male to urinate as the diameter of the prostatic urethra is reduced. Symptoms of urinary *frequency* (needing to urinate many times), urinary *hesitancy* (having difficulty beginning flow), urinary *retention* (the inability to empty the bladder), and urinary *urgency* (the feeling of needing to void immediately) are commonly associated with BPH. To observe an animated overview of BPH:

1. Click on *Clinical Animations*; Select "**All**," "**Urinary**," and "**All**" from the associated drop down menus.
2. Click "**Search**."
3. Find the animation titled *Enlarged Prostate Gland (BPH)*.

➲ Enlarged Prostate Gland (BPH)

Identify and label the components of the female urinary tract in the following figure.
To locate the image in AIA:
1. *Click on* **Atlas Anatomy**; *Select* **"Pelvis and Perineum," "Urinary," "Medial,"** *and* **"Illustration"** *from the associated drop down menus.*
2. *Click "***Search**."*
3. *Find the image titled* **Female Pelvic Organs (Med) 1**.

AA Female Pelvic Organs (Med) 1

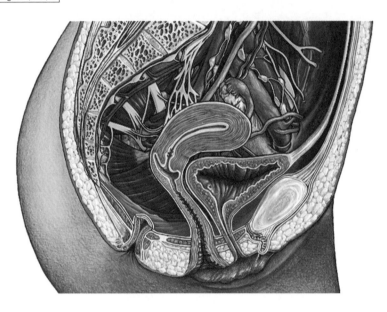

Identify and label the components of the male urinary tract in the following figure.
To locate the image in AIA:
1. *Click on* **Atlas Anatomy**; *Select* **"Pelvis and Perineum," "Urinary," "Medial,"** *and* **"Illustration"** *from the associated drop down menus.*
2. *Click "***Search**".*
3. *Find the image titled* **Male Pelvic Organs (Med) 1**.

AA Male Pelvic Organs (Med) 1

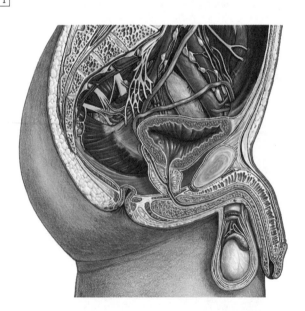

To view similar images of the female and male urinary tract you may go to **DA** ♂ MO *or* **DA** ♀ MO

URINARY SYSTEM REVIEW EXERCISES

Matching

_____ **1.** Pyramids

_____ **2.** Renal pelvis

_____ **3.** Urinary bladder

_____ **4.** Renal corpuscle

_____ **5.** Urethra

_____ **6.** Glomerulus

_____ **7.** Collecting duct

_____ **8.** Ureter

_____ **9.** Calyces

_____ **10.** Peritubular capillaries

a. consists of the glomerulus and Bowman capsule

b. carries urine from the bladder to outside the body

c. hollow spaces to collect urine from the pyramids

d. collect reabsorbed filtrate from the tubules

e. responds to hormones such as ADH and aldosterone

f. occupy the majority of the renal medulla

g. the temporary storage tank for urine

h. carries urine from the kidney to the urinary bladder

i. the capillaries responsible for filtrate formation

j. the funnel-shaped origin of the ureter

Labeling

Draw your own lines and then label the following features on the diagram.

a. Arcuate artery

b. Renal artery

c. Pyramid

d. Cortex

e. Cortical radiate artery

f. Minor calyx

g. Interlobar artery

h. Renal pelvis

i. Renal column

j. Major calyx

k. Segmental artery

l. Ureter

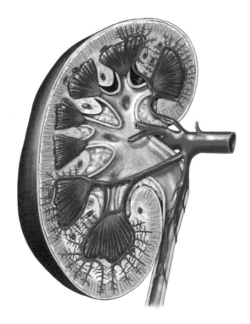

Draw your own lines and then label the following features on the diagram.

a. Arcuate artery
b. Vasa recta
c. Bowman capsule
d. Cortical radiate artery
e. Collecting duct

f. Afferent arteriole
g. Distal convoluted tubule
h. Peritubular capillaries
i. Proximal convoluted tubule
j. Efferent arteriole

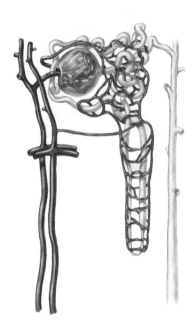

Fill in the Blank/Short Answer

1. The _____ urethral sphincter is involuntary, whereas the _____ urethral sphincter is voluntary.

2. The three divisions of the male urethra are the _____, _____, and _____.

3. The endocrine gland sitting atop of each kidney is the _____ gland.

4. The area of the bladder that is a common site for infection is the _____.

5. The urinary bladder can routinely hold as much as _____ mL of urine.

6. The hormone _____ increases the permeability of the tubule cells to water.

7. The special cells of the corpuscle with foot-like extensions are known as _____.

8. Name one reason women are more likely to suffer from urinary tract infections than men.

9. Once plasma pushes through the glomerulus and into Bowman capsule it is called _____.

10. The feeling of needing to urinate immediately is known as _____.

11. The passive force driving filtrate formation at the corpuscle is called _____.

12. The loop of _____ is made of a thin descending limb and thick ascending limb.

13. The _____ cells within the afferent arteriole help to maintain the glomerular filtration rate.

Essay

1. Trace a drop of blood from the abdominal aorta through the kidney and back to the inferior vena cava.

2. Trace a drop of urine from the renal corpuscle to outside of the body.

3. Discuss some similarities and difference between filtrate and urine.

4. Name some characteristics that make glomeruli specially designed for filtration.

Reproductive System

LEARNING OBJECTIVES

Upon completion of this chapter, the student should be able to:

Male Reproductive System

- Locate and describe the structures of the male external genitalia
- Locate and describe the accessory glands of the male reproductive system
- Locate and describe the internal anatomy of the penis and the divisions of the urethra
- Describe the pathway of sperm through the male reproductive duct system

Female Reproductive System

- Locate and describe the structures of the female external genitalia
- Locate and describe the structures of the female internal genitalia
- Describe the pathway of ova through the female reproductive duct system
- Identify the mammary gland and its associated structures

REPRODUCTIVE SYSTEM OVERVIEW

Ultimately, the role of the reproductive system is simply to propagate the human species. While almost all cells of the human body are considered *somatic* and contain 23 pairs (46 total) of chromosomes (called ***diploid*** cells), *gametes* (sperm and egg cells) contain just 23 single chromosomes and are referred to as ***haploid*** cells. Fertilization of the female egg by the male sperm allows for the development of a unique diploid *zygote*. The zygote develops into an *embryo* within the female uterus. It ultimately matures into a *fetus* until its birth after a typical 266-day gestational period. In infancy and childhood, the reproductive system is relatively dormant. Upon reaching puberty, the reproductive glands and organs are activated by pituitary hormones and begin to mature and develop in preparation for their role in creating new life.

To observe an animated, interactive overview of both conception and fetal development:
1. Click on Clinical Animations; *Select "**All**," "**Reproductive**," and "**All**" from the associated drop down menus.*
*2. Click "**Search**."*
*3. Find the animations titled **Conception - Interactive Tool** and **Fetal Development - Interactive Tool**.*

⊙ | Conception - Interactive Tool |

⊙ | Fetal Development - Interactive Tool |

LAB ACTIVITY 11.1

Male Reproductive System

The primary reproductive organs of the male are the *gonads* or **testes**. They function to both manufacture **sperm** (a process called *spermatogenesis*) and produce the hormone testosterone. Accessory organs of the male reproductive tract include several glands and ducts that produce semen and transport sperm out of the body to the female reproductive tract. The testes are housed outside of the body in a sac known as the **scrotum**. This allows the testes to remain slightly cooler than body temperature, which is necessary for normal spermatogenesis to occur. A thin layer of muscle in the scrotum known as *dartos* muscle can contract and relax, changing the size of the scrotum and helping to regulate the temperature of the testes. Cooler temperatures cause the dartos to contract, which shrinks the scrotum and moves the testes closer to the pelvis while warmer temperature allows the dartos to relax, suspending the testes a bit further from the pelvis.

To observe an animated overview of sperm production:
1. *Click on* Clinical Animations; *Select "**All**," "**Reproductive**," and "**All**" from the associated drop down menus.*
2. *Click "**Search**."*
3. *Find the animation titled **Sperm Production** and **Pathway of Ejaculation**.*

⮕ | Sperm Production and Pathway of Ejaculation |

Within each testis is a series of tubes known as seminiferous tubules where spermatogenesis actually occurs. Gametogenesis in a male (called spermatogenesis) does not begin until the age of puberty. Until that time, a boy does not manufacture any sperm. Developing sperm must therefore be kept away from the immune system so they are not recognized as "foreign." Remember, by puberty the immune system is well developed so the developing lymphocytes never had an opportunity to "see" these sperm cells in the child. From the seminiferous tubules, the immature sperm move on to the "comma-shaped" **epididymis** where they mature for a period of several weeks. Extending from the epididymis, proceeding through the inguinal canal, and arching over the superior aspect of the urinary bladder may be found the **ductus (vas) deferens**. The ductus deferens serves to transport sperm to the **ejaculatory duct**. Resting behind the posterolateral aspect of the urinary bladder are a paired set of glands known as **seminal vesicles**. The seminal vesicles produce as much as 60% of the volume of seminal fluid. Seminal fluid contains nutrients for the sperm such as fructose and vitamin C, enzymes to enhance sperm mobility, prostaglandins to help prepare the female cervix to receive the sperm, and factors to both coagulate and later liquefy the ejaculate. The seminal vesicle merges with the ductus deferens within the prostate gland to form the **ejaculatory duct**. The **prostate gland** contributes approximately one third of the volume of semen. The **bulbourethral (Cowper) glands** are the third and final glands that contribute to semen production. They are small, pea-sized glands that drain into the spongy (penile) urethra. The bulbourethral glands are activated with sexual arousal and secrete their product into the urethra *prior* to ejaculation. This pre-ejaculate is alkaline in nature and serves to remove traces of acidic urine from the urethra and also as a lubricant during sexual intercourse. Acid is generally hostile to sperm, which is why it is important for the bulbourethral secretions to cleanse the male urethra. Likewise, it is important for semen as a whole to be basic as well in order to buffer the acidic environment of the female vagina.

The **penis** is the male organ for copulation and is considered part of the external genitalia. At first glance, the penis looks singular in nature but in reality, the penis is actually made up of three distinct erectile bodies. The paired **corpora cavernosa** engorge with blood during an erection and provide the rigidity necessary to penetrate the female vagina. The singular **corpus spongiosum** engorges with arousal as well but does not assume the rigidity of the corpora cavernosa. The corpus spongiosum houses the **penile (spongy) urethra**. If it was allowed to become rigid the urethra would be compromised, preventing semen from exiting the body and thereby making eventual fertilization impossible. The corpus spongiosum terminates in an expanded tip known as the **glans penis**. At birth, the glans penis is covered by loose skin known as **prepuce**. With an erection, the prepuce retracts over the glans allowing for heightened sensitivity during intercourse. In some cultures, including many in the United States, it is common to have the prepuce surgically removed shortly after birth during a procedure known as *circumcision*.

Identify and label the male external genitalia, accessory glands, and ducts in the following figures.
To locate the lateral image in AIA:

1. *Click on **Atlas Anatomy**; Select "**Pelvis and Perineum**," "**Reproductive**," "**Lateral**," and "**Illustration**" from the associated drop down menu.*
2. *Click "**Search**."*
3. *Find the image titled **Male Pelvic Organs (Lat).***

AA Male Pelvic Organs (Lat)

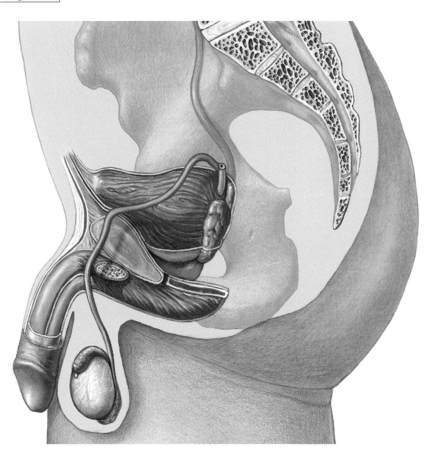

To locate the sagittal image in AIA:

1. *Click on **Atlas Anatomy**; Select "**Pelvis and Perineum**," "**Reproductive**," "**Medial**," and "**Illustration**" from the associated drop down menus.*
2. *Click "**Search**."*
3. *Find the image titled **Male Pelvic Organs (Med) 1.***

To view a similar image of the male reproductive system you may go to

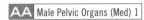

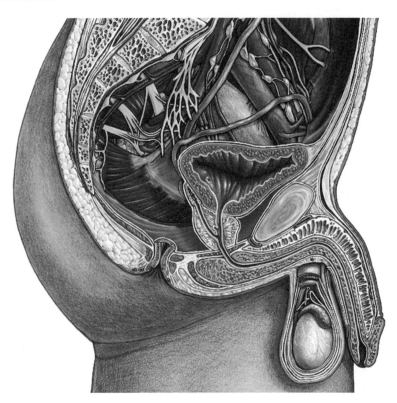

CLINICAL APPLICATIONS

A **vasectomy** is a common form of male sterilization that takes place on an outpatient basis and is typically performed in just 30 minutes. A small incision is made on either side of the scrotum to make the spermatic cord accessible. The ductus deferens is located within the spermatic cord along with various blood vessels and nerves. A small section of the ductus deferens is removed and the open ends are sealed, preventing sperm from traveling onward to the ejaculatory duct. The sperm are still manufactured however, at the rate of approximately 400 million per day, but unable to leave the body they are broken down and resorbed with the help of macrophages. With varying degrees of success, some vasectomies may be reversed but the procedure is designed to be a permanent form of sterilization.

To observe an animated overview of a vasectomy:
1. *Click on Clinical Animations; Select "**All**," "**Reproductive**," and "**All**" from the associated drop down menus.*
2. *Click "**Search**."*
3. *Find the animation titled **Vasectomy**.*

Vasectomy

CI Pathway of Sperm

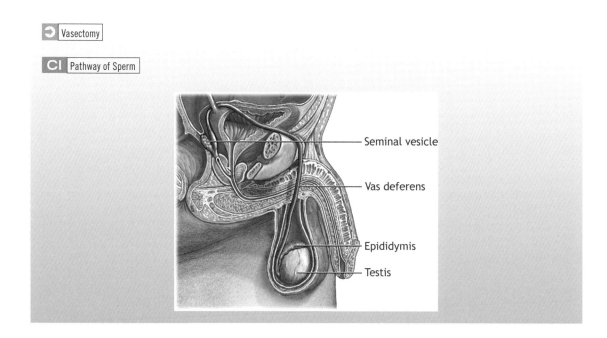

- Seminal vesicle
- Vas deferens
- Epididymis
- Testis

*For a unique interactive experience and a different view of the male reproductive system click on the **3D Anatomy** icon and then select **3D Male Reproductive System**.*

3D Male Reproductive System

From there, you are able to manipulate a 3D recreation by rotating it, moving it, zooming in and out, and even experience cut-away views.

LAB ACTIVITY 11.2

Female Reproductive System

The primary reproductive organs of the female are the *gonads* or **ovaries**. They function to both manufacture **ova** or **eggs** (a process called *oogenesis*) and produce the hormones estrogen and progesterone. Accessory organs of the female reproductive tract serve to receive semen from the male; allow for fertilization, transportation, and implantation of the ovum; and nourish the developing fetus. The ovaries, unlike the male testes, are housed within the pelvic cavity. Also unlike the male, gametogenesis in a female (called oogenesis) occurs before birth. A female is born with all of the eggs she will ever have (~2 million of them). They remain dormant until puberty when they are stimulated to mature with the cyclic release of sex hormones from the anterior pituitary gland.

To observe an animated overview of egg cell production:
*1. Click on **Clinical Animations**; Select "**All**," "**Reproductive**," and "**All**" from the associated drop down menus*
*2. Click "**Search**"*
*3. Find the animation titled **Egg Cell Production***

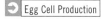 Egg Cell Production

Upon ovulation, the ovum is ejected from the ovary and then gets swept into the **uterine (Fallopian) tube** by finger-like extensions of the tube known as **fimbriae**. It is important to note that there is no actual physical connection between the ovary and uterine tube. The uterine tube is the actual site of fertilization of the egg by the sperm and failure of the egg to be swept into the tube after ovulation may lead to an *ectopic* pregnancy (a pregnancy that occurs outside of the uterus). The uterine tubes course proximally toward the uterus and enter at its superolateral aspect. The region of the uterus above the entrance of the uterine tubes is known as the **fundus**. The uterus is a thick, muscular organ that serves as the womb, allowing for the development and maturation of the fetus. The outer layer is consistent with the peritoneum and is known as the **perimetrium**. The thick, middle layer is called the **myometrium**. The inner layer is known as the **endometrium**. It is this endometrium that prepares itself every month to receive a fertilized ovum. If a fertilized ovum reaches the endometrial wall, it will implant into the uterine lining where it will be nourished by endometrial glands until the placenta forms. If an unfertilized ovum reaches the uterus levels of estrogen and progesterone will sharply fall, causing the endometrial lining to be sloughed off and shed as menses. This regular, cyclic regeneration, preparation, and eventual sloughing off of the endometrial lining lasts roughly 28 days and is known as the *menstrual cycle*.

To observe an animated, interactive overview of the menstrual cycle:
1. *Click on **Clinical Animations**; Select "**All**," "**Reproductive**," and "**All**" from the associated drop down menus.*
2. *Click "**Search**."*
3. *Find the animation titled **Menstrual Cycle - Interactive Tool**.*

➲ | Menstrual Cycle - Interactive Tool

CLINICAL APPLICATIONS

A **Pap smear** is a test that involves scraping the outer lining of the cervix to remove some cells. These cells are then looked at under a microscope to determine if there are any cancerous or abnormal (**dysplastic**) cells that may be likely to turn into **cervical cancer**. Pap smears are routinely performed on women over the age of 21 during their annual visit to the Ob/Gyn. **Dilation and curettage (D&C)** is a procedure where the cervix is dilated (opened) and a special instrument called a curette is inserted through the cervix into the uterine cavity. The inner uterine lining is then scraped away and collected for examination. A D&C may be performed to remove small pieces of the placenta after childbirth or to remove uterine tissue after a miscarriage. D&Cs may also help diagnose problems associated with heavy menstrual bleeding such as **endometriosis**, **fibroids**, or uterine cancer.

To view additional images of the cervix, Pap smear, D&C, and endometriosis in AIA:
1. *Click on "Clinical Illustrations"; Select "**Pelvis and Perineum**," "**Reproductive**," "**All**," "**All**," and "**Obstetrics and Gynecology (OB/GYN)**" from the associated drop down menus.*
2. *Click "Search."*
3. *Find the corresponding images.*

The inferior aspect of the uterus actually extends downward into the vaginal canal as a thickened muscular region known as the **cervix**. The cervix contains the narrow **cervical canal** with its outer opening, the **external os**, facing the vagina and its inner opening, the **internal os**, facing the inside of the uterine body. The **vagina** is the female organ of copulation, which receives the penis during coitis or sexual intercourse. In addition to its copulatory role, the vagina also serves as the birth canal as well as the route for the elimination of monthly menses from the body. The vagina is approximately 3.5 inches in length and extends from the vestibule (outside the body) to the uterus, internally. There is space between the vaginal wall and the cervix, known as the **fornix**, which can expand to receive the glans penis during intercourse. From a frontal section, you may view the lateral fornices, whereas a sagittal section will show the anterior and posterior fornices.

The vagina opens to become part of the external genitalia at the opening of the vestibule. From anterior to posterior, the vestibule contains the clitoris, urethral orifice, and vaginal orifice. The **clitoris** is homologous to the male glans penis, containing erectile tissue and housing the greatest abundance of sensitive nerve endings. Lateral to the vaginal orifice are a pair of thin folds of mucosa known as **labia minora**. Anteriorly the labia minora unite to form a hood or **prepuce**, which covers over the clitoris. With arousal the clitoris will engorge with blood allowing it to slightly protrude from this prepuce. A fatty pad of tissue known as the **mons pubis** overlies the pubic symphysis. The mons pubis cushions and protects the pubic bone, especially during intercourse. Extending posterior and inferior from the mons pubis are a pair of thick, hair-covered folds known as **labia majora**. Developmentally, the labia majora are homologous to the male scrotum. In a normal, nonaroused state, the labia majora encase the smaller, more medial labia minora, which in turn cover over the vestibule. At birth, a female is born with a thin, perforated mucosal membrane, the **hymen**, blocking the entrance to the vagina. The hymen helps prevent the entrance of nondesirable substances into the vagina while the perforations allow for the flow of menses to leave the body prior to the time of first coitis. This vascular membrane will typically bleed a bit at the time of its initial rupture: typically with the initial encounter of sexual intercourse, the first use of a tampon, or even sometimes as a result of a strenuous sports-type activity.

Identify and label the visible female external genitalia, vagina, uterus, uterine tubes, and ovaries in the following figure.

To locate the lateral image in AIA:

1. *Click on **Atlas Anatomy**; Select "**Pelvis and Perineum**," "**Reproductive**," "**Lateral**," and "**Illustration**" from the associated drop down menus.*
2. *Click "**Search**."*
3. *Find the image titled **Female Pelvic Organs (Lat)**.*

AA Female Pelvic Organs (Lat)

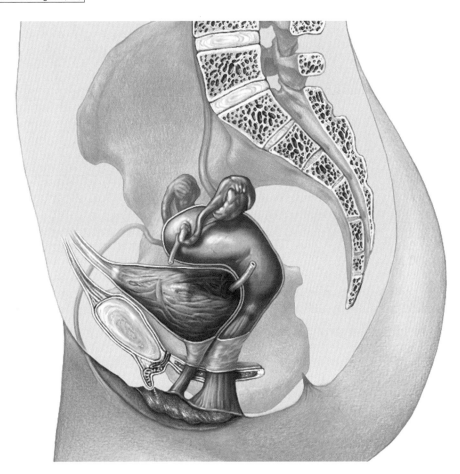

To locate the sagittal image in AIA:

1. *Click on **Atlas Anatomy**; Select "**Pelvis and Perineum**," "**Reproductive**," "**Medial**," and "**Illustration**" from the associated drop down menus.*
2. *Click "**Search**."*
3. *Find the image titled **Male Pelvic Organs (Med) 1**.*

To view a similar image of the male reproductive system you may go to

AA Female Pelvic Organs (Med) 1

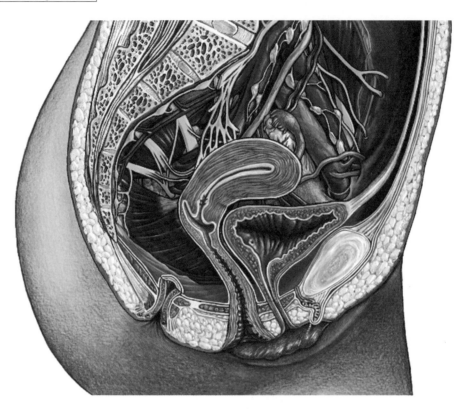

CLINICAL APPLICATIONS

Remember that …the vagina is open to the outside…and the cervix is open to both the vagina and uterus…and the uterus is open to the fallopian tubes, and the fallopian tubes do not touch the ovaries so therefore open directly into the pelvic cavity. Some sexually transmitted diseases (STDs) such as chlamydia are considered "silent" diseases because many of those individuals who are infected do not present with any symptoms. Left untreated, an infection can spread through the cervix and uterine tubes into the pelvic cavity. When scarring occurs in the pelvic cavity, it can lead to chronic pain and inflammation known as ***pelvic inflammatory disease*** (PID). In some cases, once the "painless" infection and scarring has occurred throughout the uterine tubes, it may lead to infertility in the woman. Glands within the cervix produce a thickened mucus that blocks the external os for the majority of the menstrual cycle, specifically to keep what is introduced into the vagina from spreading internally. However, in the five days or so surrounding the time of ovulation the cervical mucus thins and becomes less viscous to allow for easier entry of the sperm and semen into the uterus in hopes of fertilizing the ovum.

For a unique interactive experience and a better view of the female external genitalia click on the **3D Anatomy** *icon and then select* **3D Female Reproductive System**.

3D Female Reproductive System

From there you are able to manipulate a three-dimensional recreation by rotating it, moving it, zooming in and out, and even experience cut-away views.

LAB ACTIVITY 11.3

Mammary Glands

While both males and females have **mammary glands** present, they are generally only functional in the female. The female breasts are stimulated to increase in size and function with the increase in female sex hormones around the time of puberty. The sole role of the mammary glands is to provide nourishment via the production of breast milk, called *lactation*. Internally, each breast is divided into a collection of 20 or so **lobes** that are arranged around the central nipple, similar to the arrangement of spokes on a tire. Each lobe contains smaller **lobules,** which are just clusters of glandular **alveoli**, or sacs, that produce milk during lactation. Each lobe contains a **lactiferous duct** that carries the milk toward the **nipple**. These ducts open into a slightly larger space, just deep to the darkened circle around the nipple known as the **areola**. The spaces themselves are known as **lactiferous sinuses**, which function to hold a small amount of milk while nursing. The lobes of the breast are separated from each other by connective tissue (*suspensory ligaments*) and adipose tissue. It is important to remember that generally speaking, the variation in the sizes of different breasts has more to do with the amount of adipose tissue than the amount of glandular tissue. Large breasts do not necessarily produce more milk. Even a smaller-sized breast should be able to adequately supply enough milk to sustain an infant through breast feeding.

Identify and label the features of the mammary glands in the following figures. To view the anterior image in AIA, go to

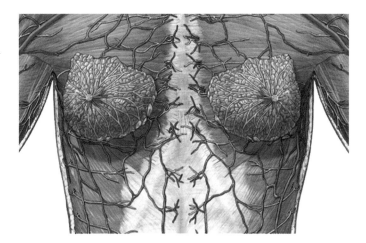

To view the sagittal image in AIA, go to

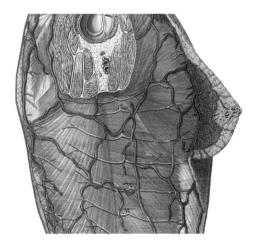

CLINICAL APPLICATIONS

A **mammogram** is an x-ray image of the breast. The two major types of mammograms are *screening mammograms* that are performed as a preventive measure to check for breast cancer in women with no signs and symptoms. A *diagnostic mammogram* is performed to check for breast cancer after a lump or some other sign or symptom of breast cancer has already been discovered. There is some controversy in the health care community about who should receive mammograms and at what age. Some organizations recommend screenings to begin at age 40 while others feel it is more appropriate to wait until age 50. Some recommend screenings annually while others feel every 2 to 3 years is sufficient. While the amount of radiation exposure is quite low with each mammogram, repeated exposure to x-rays can be problematic for some. Mammography is occasionally associated with *false-positive* results—that is, the radiologist believes the test is positive for breast cancer but in fact there is no cancer present. This often causes a great deal of anxiety and stress in the patient. False-negative results also occur on occasion—meaning breast cancer is actually present although it cannot be seen on the mammogram. *False-negative* tests occur at a higher rate in women with more dense breasts and therefore occur more frequently in younger women. It is important for a woman to discuss the benefits and risks of mammography with her physician to come up with a plan that is most appropriate. It is also important that a woman receives instruction on how to perform a **self-breast exam**. These exams may be performed on a monthly basis and should involve both a visual and manual inspection to detect any changes in contour, texture, or density of the breast tissue. Self-breast exams are quick, easy, and may be performed in the privacy of one's home.

To view a few images of breast anatomy, breast lumps, breast cancer, and mammography in AIA:

4. *Click on "Clinical Illustrations"; Select "**Thorax**," "**Reproductive**," "**All**," "**All**," and "**Obstetrics** and **Gynecology (OB/GYN)**" from the associated drop down menus*
5. *Click "**Search**"*
6. *Find the corresponding images*

REPRODUCTIVE SYSTEM REVIEW EXERCISES

Matching

_____ **1.** Epididymis

_____ **2.** Membranous urethra

_____ **3.** Prostate gland

_____ **4.** Corpora cavernosa

_____ **5.** Prepuce

_____ **6.** Scrotum

_____ **7.** Seminal vesicle

_____ **8.** Bulbourethral gland

_____ **9.** Ejaculatory duct

_____ **10.** Corpus spongiosum

a. covers the glans penis

b. produces 1/3 of seminal fluid

c. the sac containing the testes

d. secretes a lubricating pre-ejaculate

e. produces 60% of seminal fluid

f. erectile tissue containing majority of urethra

g. storage site for immature sperm

h. located within the prostate gland

i. paired erectile tissue responsible for rigidity

j. passes through the urogenital diaphragm

Matching

_____ **1.** Hymen

_____ **2.** Fimbriae

_____ **3.** Uterus

_____ **4.** External os

_____ **5.** Ovary

_____ **6.** Clitoris

_____ **7.** Vagina

_____ **8.** Mons pubis

_____ **9.** Labia majora

_____ **10.** Prepuce

a. contains abundant sensitive nerve endings

b. paired structures found guarding the vestibule

c. site of oogenesis

d. birth canal

e. finger-like extensions of the uterine tube

f. hood over the clitoris formed by union of labia minora

g. perforated membrane guarding the vaginal orifice

h. site of implantation of fertilized egg

i. outer opening of cervical canal

j. fat pad cushioning the pubic symphysis

Labeling

Draw your own lines and then label the following features on the diagram.

a.	Corpus spongiosum	**g.**	Prostatic urethra
b.	Epididymis	**h.**	Seminal vesicle
c.	Glans penis	**i.**	Penile urethra
d.	Ejaculatory duct	**j.**	Prostate gland
e.	Corpus cavernosum	**k.**	Vas deferens
f.	Testis	**l.**	Membranous urethra

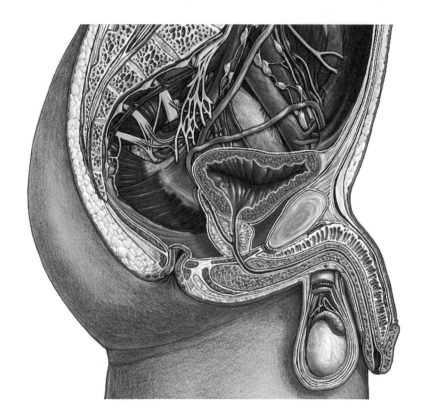

Draw your own lines and then label the following features on the diagram.

a. Vagina

b. Ovary

c. Clitoris

d. Mons pubis

e. Fimbriae

f. Labia minora

g. Myometrium

h. Posterior fornix

i. Urethra

j. Cervical canal

k. Uterine tube

l. Labia majora

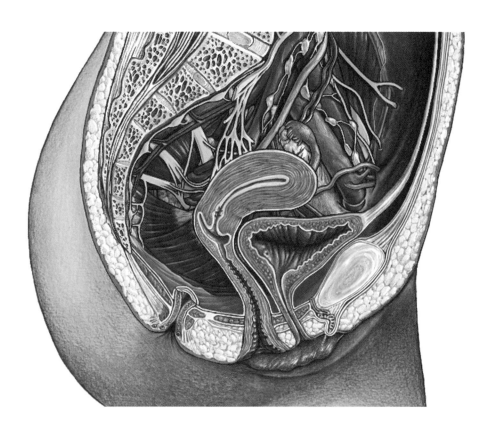

Fill in the Blank/Short Answer

1. The chief hormone secreted by the testes is _____.

2. The surgical removal of the prepuce in a male is known as _____.

3. The ejaculatory duct is formed by the union of the _____ and the

   _____.

4. The 3 glands that contribute to seminal fluid production are the _____,

   _____, and _____.

5. The duct responsible for transporting sperm from the epididymis is the _____.

6. The three erectile bodies of the penis include the paired corpora _____ and the

   single corpus _____

7. The perforated membrane protecting the vagina in a child is the _____.

8. The lining of the uterus that is shed with monthly menses is known as a _____.

9. The female structure homologous to the male glans penis is the _____.

10. The production of sperm is known as _____ while egg production is referred to as

    _____.

11. The average menstrual cycle lasts _____ days.

12. A pregnancy that occurs outside of the uterine cavity is known as an _____

    pregnancy.

13. A STD that makes its way into the pelvic cavity may lead to a painful condition called

    _____ _____ _____.

Essay

1. Describe the pathway of sperm from their production site to the site of fertilization of the ovum.

2. Describe the composition of semen and include the glands that contribute to its formation.

3. Describe the external genitalia of the female and discuss the orientation of the three major openings
    in the area.